PHARMACOLOGY - RESEARCH, SAFETY TESTING AND REGULATION

OPTIMIZATION OF DRUG PRESCRIBING IN ELDERLY

PHARMACOLOGY - RESEARCH, SAFETY TESTING AND REGULATION

Additional books in this series can be found on Nova's website under the Series tab.

Additional e-books in this series can be found on Nova's website under the e-book tab.

PHARMACOLOGY - RESEARCH, SAFETY TESTING AND REGULATION

OPTIMIZATION OF DRUG PRESCRIBING IN ELDERLY

HUGO JUÁREZ OLGUÍN
AND
ISMAEL LARES ASSEFF
EDITORS

nova publishers
New York

Library of Congress Cataloging-in-Publication Data

ISBN: 978-1-63484-879-4

Library of Congress Control Number: 2016933386

Published by Nova Science Publishers, Inc. † New York

CONTENTS

PREFACE

AGING, CLINICAL PHARMACOKINETIC AND PERSONALIZED PHARMACOTHERAPY

Aging process begins right from the birth of an individual and continues all through the life and as growth and development progress in conformity with the advance of age, maturity is reached and finally senescence or old age. This stage is characterized by important biological, biochemical and physiological changes that occur in line with different life styles and nutritional changes particular to this age which is characterized by reduced physical activity and increase in chronic degenerative diseases that demand multiple uses of drugs. Within this uninterrupted process that lingers all through the life, changes in body mass growth (physical growth with anthropometrical changes) continues to take place as well as the complexity of its functions (development). Both processes gradually progress to maturity and then begin to progressively decline during senescence.

The processes leading to "growth-development-maturity-aging" imply changes in the biological, physiological and biochemical composition of the organism which continues to transpire as their complexity advances (as they progress in complexity). In the first years of life, the percentages of total body fluid as well as intra and extra cellular fluid are very elevated in childhood. These percentages keep on reducing during the process of growth and development and culminate to aging. So, in such a way that as the people get older, the percentage of body fluid continues to decreases and the percentage of fat increases and this tendency is continued until senescence.

Such changes in the biochemical composition of the organism become more evident in senescence with predominance of body fat, a situation that favors the accumulation and slow elimination of liposoluble drugs and a decrease in apparent volume of distribution for liposoluble drugs. Such aging process carries with it biological changes not only in the organic levels but also in the functional aspects which would influence in a very important form on the kinetic processes of drug absorption, distribution, metabolism and excretion (LADME system).

All these changes would modify the pharmacokinetics and pharmacodynamics of drugs which the people older than 60 years are exposed to, since their predisposition to suffer a greater number of diseases particular to this life stage makes them to require many drugs and hence predisposes them to polypharmacy which carries with it the susceptibility to present pharmacokinetic and/or pharmacodynamic interactions and consequently, more tendency to suffer adverse events to the drugs.

As the people progress in their age, their physical capacities and abilities tends downward, and their recent memory decreases. In line with the above, are higher predisposition to suffer complex and chronic degenerative diseases, partial or total anodontia, reduced or disorders of vision, benign prosthetic hypertrophy, higher predisposition to present urinary tract infection and respiratory diseases among others. All these diseases predispose people more than 60 years old to drug dependency. The majority of pharmacokinetic studies have been carried out in healthy adults, particularly those focused on clinical phase for the development of new medicines, but only few were centered on senescent individuals, in such a way that the application of the pharmacokinetic and pharmacodynamic criteria on hospitalized senescent patients with different pathologies are scanty, especially in latinamerican countries where a greater attention is required in this population sector.

In spite of the fact that senescent people are considered as individuals with high risk of intoxication and therapeutic failure especially when the therapeutic schemes used in adults are applied to them, the application of clinical pharmacokinetic and drug monitorization are not routine practice. This risk even becomes untold when talking of high risk drugs as those with narrow therapeutic index or when various drugs used at the same time as it is in the case of polypharmacy.

An important aspect, which has not been much taken into account in latinamerican countries, is personalized drug-therapy that considers the importance of inter and intra-individual variabilities demonstrated in pharmacokinetic studies and more recently, in the contributions of pharmacogenetics, disciplines that have put into evidence the inter-ethnic differences in the response to treatment and whose aspects, for being new knowledge, ought to be taken into consideration so as to bring to practice a personalized medicine and pharmacokinetic in geriatric patients. Presently, the dosification and the establishment of therapeutic scheme ought to be based on pharmacokinetic, pharmacodynamic and pharmacogenetic knowledge with special emphasis on the exclusive characteristics of senescent individuals.

Ismael Lares Asseff

In: Optimization of Drug Prescribing in Elderly ISBN: 978-1-63484-879-4
Editors: Juárez O. H. and Lares A. I. © 2016 Nova Science Publishers, Inc.

Chapter 1

WHAT IS THERAPEUTIC OPTIMIZATION SCHEDULE OF DRUGS USED IN ELDERLY?

Ismael Lares Asseff*

Centro Interdisciplinario de Investigación para el Desarrollo Integral Regional (CIIDIR), Instituto Politécnico Nacional, Durango, México

ABSTRACT

Therapeutic optimization of drugs in clinical practice is required for improving and assuring the efficacy and safety of drugs. The development process of a new drug comprises the preclinical phase, carried out *in vitro* and in animal models; and the clinical phase, done for the first time in human beings. The later consists of four phases – I, II, III, and IV, and the primary objective is to guarantee to the maximum, the reduction of risk of presenting adverse events and/or therapeutic failure.

The process of aging is a fundamental part of growth and development. From biological, physiological and pharmacological point of views, the final stage of this process is fraught with exceptional characteristics that keep on modifying due to changes peculiar to senescence. For this, pharmacological and therapeutic managements in the elderly need to be based on a careful approach in which all these inherent changes as well as interindividual variabilities have to be considered. Studies carried out in youths and old aged people have shown

* Corresponding autor: Ismael Lares Asseff, Instituto Politécnico Nacional, CIIDIR-Unidad Durango, Calle Sigma 119. Fracc. 20 de noviembre II, Durango. Durango, Mexico, C.P. 34220. E-mail: ismaelares@ yahoo.com.

that these peculiar changes in senescence make the elderly a risk group prone to intoxication and/or therapeutic failure. For this reason, it is obligatory to know the particular pharmacokinetic and pharmacodynamic changes on the basis of age range and the processes of disease development in aged people which often have a link to these special characteristics.

Given that the life expectancy has continued to increase in the last years in countries like Mexico, the population of individuals over 60 years old has notably gone up in latinamerican countries. This has resulted in a greater demand for drug consumption, especially those employed in the management of ailments that form part of aging process. In occasions, the people in this age population practice polypharmacy with its concomitant pharmacokinetic and pharmacodynamic interactions with important repercussions from clinical point of view and pharmaco-economic implications. For the above, we propose the necessity to promote the program of therapeutic drug optimization in geriatric population.

INTRODUCTION

The most used program of drug optimization in pediatric and geriatrics was established based on the objective to improve the effectiveness and safety of drugs frequently used in individuals over 60 years. The creation of the National Institute of Science and Technology for Child Health in 1976 by the Mexican Institution for Child Welfare (IMAN) has as its principal objective to perform and promote scientific research and technological development suitable for solving health problems in the field of pediatrics. In 1982, the National System for Integral Family Development (DIF), based on the National Development Plan (in the area of health), established in INCYTAS-DIF program the Optimization of Medication therapies that are most used in geriatrics and pediatrics, thus making children and elderly people the main groups of study.

Upon the approval of the Law on National Social Assistance System in January 1985, proposed by the DIF, and based on Articles 3, 4 and 11 (in their sections II and VIII) of this Act, a greater support from the DIF to this program with human and technical resources for its development came into effect.

The Institute of Scientific Investigation of Juarez University of the State of Durango through the Training Program and Promotion of Human Resources Research, established a collaborative agreement with the National Institute of

Sciences and Technologies for Health-DIF in 1988, in order to conduct scientific studies with the acquisition of knowledge for the planning of final solutions to priority health problems and social assistance.

Among the priorities defined by the two institutions were to conduct original scientific research on problems of health and social care at national level in - DIF population System. The characteristics of this population are generally poor, vulnerable, physical and mental handicap, children, adolescents, pregnant women, disabled and elderly people.

As a result of collaborative efforts between the two institutions, this monograph was prepared with the aim of showing the results of the research on "Geriatric Pharmacology," and to provide original and up-to-date knowledge on rational use of drugs in a sector of the population which has not been given the due social importance, even when this is increasingly evident in the aging processes which is the final part of the process of human growth and development, and as a population that is growing not only in our country but also in the world.

Expanding the coverage of care and research in senescence is of vital importance because people over 60 years old represent a population at high risk of intoxication and/or therapeutic inefficiency, when they are put in the same treatment regimens as in younger individuals where such regime might be efficient.

To determine the causes and mechanisms of therapeutic failure in the elderly, it is important to consider some factors marking the characteristic of old age. These factors include:

1. Changes in biological, physiological and chemical compositions associated with increasing age that produce changes in the pharmacokinetics and pharmacodynamics of drugs in these people and
2. The importance this population from the point of view of healthcare. In developed countries like the United States this population constitutes 11% of the general population, and consumes 25% of all prescription and non-prescription drugs [1].

In the case of Mexico, although the percentage of people over 60 years is not as high as in the case of developed countries. In 1980, this population only accounted for 5.7% of the total population. However, in absolute terms, the increase has been very significant since the early 50's. In the period from 1970 to the year 2000, the total population increased on average annual rate of 2.4%

while the group over 60 years old was 3.2%. In 1970, the population of people older than 60 years was 2.7 million and in 2000, it increase to 6.9 million and with this, the proportion of aged adults passed from 5.6% to 7.1% in this lapse of time. According to the predictive calculations of the Mexican National Population Board, it is expected that for the year 2025, the proportion of the people over 60 years old will be 25% and for 2050, this will be about 28% [2]. These observations are very important when the impact on healthcare demand and social assistance to this segment of population is considered. To improve the health and therefore quality of life of elderly, DIF (INCYTAS) conducted a research aimed at optimizing the therapeutic drug management for drugs of frequent use in geriatrics with emphasis on the knowledge of the pharmacokinetics of the same, and their relationship with their peculiar biological changes of aging, which will allow a more rational therapeutic management of medicines prescribed by the doctors. Also, such research is intended to provide a guide to avoid the abuse of medical prescriptions, self-medication, noncompliance, drug interactions and to improve drug-surveillance.

The primary objective of the program of optimizing therapeutic drugs most widely used in geriatrics was to study the pharmacokinetics of the drugs under the living conditions of Mexican elderly people.

The goals to be achieved were:

1. To increase the knowledge on the pharmacokinetics of drugs in order to establish appropriate dosing regimens.
2. To evaluate the efficacy and safety of treatment regimens based on the pharmacokinetic knowledge of mostly used drugs.
3. To establish pharmacokinetic data based on different drugs in different populations and with different biological characteristics, which can be used in clinical practice. Likewise, we hope that these data can be reused to validate future mathematical models and/or pharmacokinetic predictive models and simulation.
4. To establish a drug-monitoring program for drugs with high toxicity index and/or narrow therapeutic range. Also, to identify and monitor drug levels in individuals at risk of intoxication or treatment failure.
5. To train the clinicians and health staffs on pharmacokinetic applications in the clinics at the three levels of health care in the country.

REFERENCES

[1] Fialová D. and Onder G., "Medication errors in elderly people: contributing factors and future perspectives.," *Br. J. Clin. Pharmacol.*, vol. 67, no. 6, pp. 641-5, Jun. 2009.

[2] Guzmán B. and U. S. B. of the Census, *The Hispanic population, 2000*, Volume 8, Issue 2. U.S. Dept. of Commerce, Economics and Statistics Administration, U.S. Census Bureau, 2001.

In: Optimization of Drug Prescribing in Elderly ISBN: 978-1-63484-879-4
Editors: Juárez O. H. and Lares A. I.

Chapter 2

OVERVIEW OF THE COMMON GERIATRIC ILLNESS

Stephanie Rubi Pérez Saldaña *
and Diego Zamora de la Cruz
Departamento de Farmacología, Facultad de Medicina,
Universidad Nacional Autónoma de Mexico, Mexico City, Mexico

ABSTRACT

Aging is a physiological process that is characterized by cessation of body functions. However, aging is not synonymous of disease. People who are over 60 years old are considered to be senior citizens and currently in the world, the population of elderly people is put to approximately 420 millions. Adult people with this age and above undergo a series of physiological changes that make them vulnerable to suffer a wide range of diseases in different organs of the body. Among such diseases, we can pinpoint ailments like visual impairment, hearing loss, cardiovascular problems, diabetes, dementia, and Parkinson disease. Physiological changes produce alteration in drug metabolism the consequence of which may be greater adverse effects and thus, polypharmacy. In this population, the main causes of death are neoplasia, cardiovascular and complications of chronic diseases. It is therefore

* Corresponding author: Stephanie Rubi Pérez Saldaña; Departamento de Farmacología, Universidad Nacional Autónoma de México; Ciudad Universitaria, CP 04130, Mexico City, Mexico; e-mail: rubimode@hotmail.com.

pertinent to point out that a good management of geriatric patients should begin with comprehensive and multifactorial studies to dig out all the etiological facts of their ailments that would enable the right decision of approaches which would grant welfare with good quality of life to them. This chapter takes a comprehensive look at the evaluation of geriatric patients, the principal morbidities and their treatments.

INTRODUCTION

Aging is a process that varies from one individual to another and occurs as a natural effect of time and sometimes, it is accompanied by deteriorations of some physiological functions. This process, by itself, is not necessarily associated to a disease or illness. Nonetheless, during the process, such ailments like hearing impairment, motor and visual problems among others are eminent and these can lead to a loss of independence by the elderly person, a situation that can aggravate the diseases commonly associated with aging [1]. The velocity of this process depends on the life expectancy, causes of morbidity and mortality in the general population.

According to WHO (World Health Organization) [2, 3], aging can be considered as a success of public health policies, socioeconomic developments and the willingness to assume the challenges to improve the health and functional capacity of older adults.

The onset of notable deficits in functionality in the people begins when they are over 60 years old, an age they are taken to be elder people, however, not seen as sick individuals. Geriatric patients, apart from having the same physiological characteristics, differ from elder people by undergoing through numerous diseases that subject them to dependency and hence high social and economic cost to their families and the society in general. The management of this kind of people should be in the hand of specialists (the geriatricians) [2].

EPIDEMIOLOGY

According to the criteria of ONU, aging in a given population takes place when more than 5% of the population is $\geq$ 65 years old, or more than 10% is $\geq$60 years old. This is an important indicator for planning the governmental distribution of resources, since in the future more of these resources should be dedicated for the care of these people in terms of facilities, medicines and health staff [3].

Currently, there are more than 420 million older people in the world. Today in Mexico, there are about 7% of people with 60 or more years old. This means that Mexico ranks seventh among countries with accelerated aging [4]. It is projected that by 2025, this phenomenon will witness a significant increase and that more than 12% of the world population will be represented by people over 60 years old.

It is interesting to note based on these epidemiological facts that the provenance of 70% of this population is in developing countries. Such projection is substantiated based on the calculation that by 2025, the life expectancy will increase to 72 years. Due to the increase in the life expectancy, the rising low birth rate, and individual and governmental efforts to lengthen the years of healthy life of the people through adequate health care, efforts termed as intensification of the process of aging, it is expected that by 2050 one in every four Mexicans will be more than 60 years old. This will definitely impose different problems with great socio-structural, economic and environmental impacts as well as health implications rooted in an increase in chronic degenerative diseases, such as diabetes, cardiovascular diseases, hypertension and cancer [4, 5].

Originally and in descending order of incidence, these go from accidents, infectious diseases to parasitosis and subsequently chronic degenerative diseases. These pathologies lead to gradual loss of physical and social skills that ultimately end in death in these patients [6].

The most common diseases of the elderly people are heart diseases, tumors, diabetes, accidents and cirrhosis, all with diverse etiology [6]. Other diseases associated with age are trauma, malnutrition, visual diseases like cataract and glaucoma that may lead to loss of vision as well as complications of diabetes which do not cause direct death by themselves but can provoke severe disabilities. Furthermore, the psychiatric disorders like dementia and depression are very important in this age. The drugs occupied in their treatment can cause a number of undesirable effects in the elderly people and such effects can lead to serious systemic disturbances. In addition, alcoholism and some drugs addictively consumed to cope with certain terminal diseases constitute problems of addiction that these people can suffer.

In Mexico, the population health situation depends on several factors among which are age, social risks and access to health services. The youths, i.e., people in the age of growth and development, enjoy better health condition. On the contrary, social risks like alcoholism, smoking, bulimia or malnutrition conditions deteriorate the health of the people. The 1999 mortality survey in Mexico showed that the principal cause of death in older people were chronic pulmonary obstructive disease, cardiac, cerebrovascular, metabolic and malignant diseases (Table 1) [7].

Table 1. Main causes of death by sex in the elderly in México, 1999

Men	Women
1. Chronic Pulmonary Obstructive Disease (49.6%)	1. Cerebrovascular disease (40.8%)
2. Cardiac diseases (34.4%)	2. Cardiac diseases (39.0%)
3. Malignancies (29.0%)	3. Chronic Pulmonary Obstructive Disease (37.4%)
4. Diabetes mellitus (24.5%)	4. Diabetes mellitus (34.3%)
5. Cerebro-vascular disease (12.7%)	5. Malignancies (25.7%)

Mortality 1999, SSA/México.

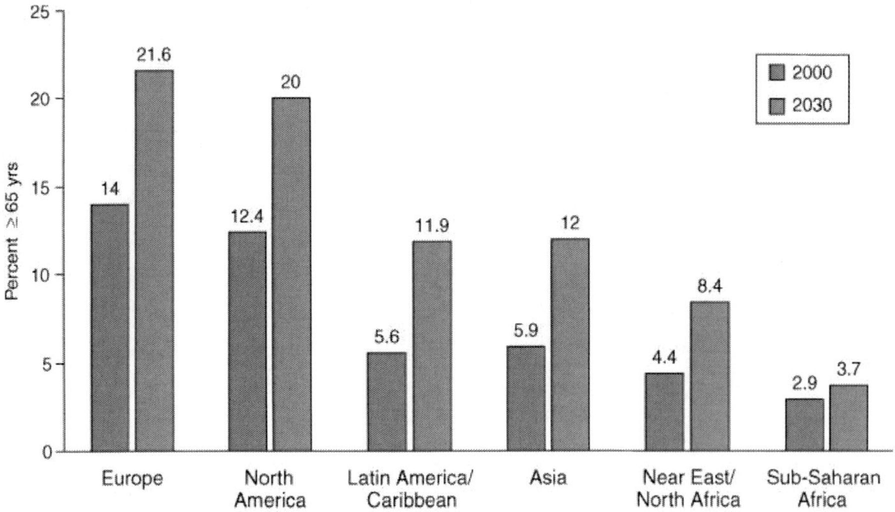

Source: Halter JB, Ouslander JG, Tinetti ME, Studenski S, High KP, Asthana S: Hazzard's Geriatric Medicine and Gerontology, 6th Edition: http://www.accessmedicine.com.

Figure 1. Percentage of senior citizens in 2000 and their estimated percentage in 2030.

The percentage of older adults in 2000 census and the projected estimated percentage for 2030 do not only show that this tendency is increasing but also disease prevalence in this group of the population (Figure 2). This implies an increase in morbidity in this group. The implication is that in future, Mexico will need more trained physicians who are not only capable of distinguishing the leading cause of morbidity and mortality in older people but also proficient in designing the right therapeutic approach and tool for the management of this group of population (Figure 1) [6].

Clinic Features of the Diseases in Elderly People

Aging involves numerous mental, psychosocial and physiological changes that increase the risk of developing a pathology. Because of the extensive nature of diseases of the elderly people, in this chapter, we will give a brief description of the most common ones and for better understanding and simplicity, the topic is approached in two big groups:

- The geriatric syndromes, and
- Specific pathologies by organs and systems.

Geriatric Syndromes

The term "Geriatric Syndromes" refers to some conditions that cause a deleterious effect on the function and quality of life of elderly people characterized by a multifactorial pathophysiology involving organs and systems outside the apparent complaint of the patient with typical clinical manifestations [8]. Within these syndromes, we can highlight frailty, falls, dizziness, syncope, pressure, ulcers, delirium, incontinence and sleep disorder [9].

A reference to Figure 2 depicts the relationship between risk factors and geriatric syndromes. The pivot of all these syndromes is the syndrome of frailty which might lead the patient to death if untreated.

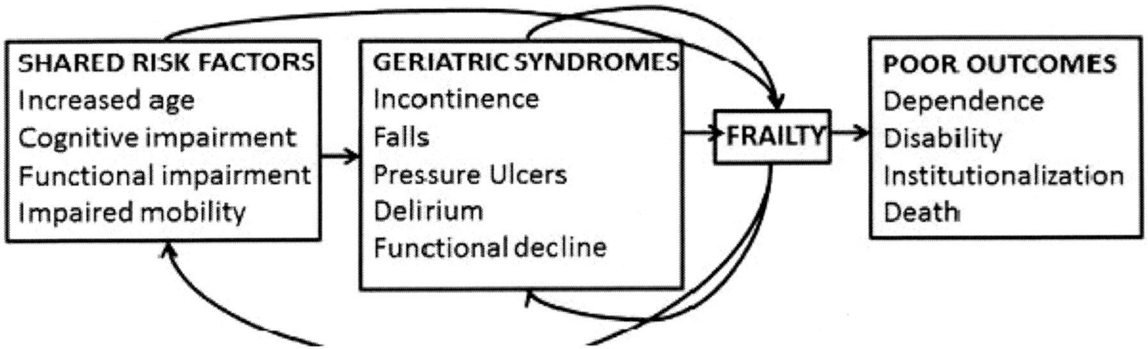

(Adapted from Inouye SK, Studenski S, Tinetti ME, et al. Geriatric Syndromes: clinical, research, and policy implications of a core geriatric concept. *J Am Geriatr Soc* 2007; 55:782; with permission) [8].

Figure 2. Relationship between risk factors, geriatric syndromes and poor performance.

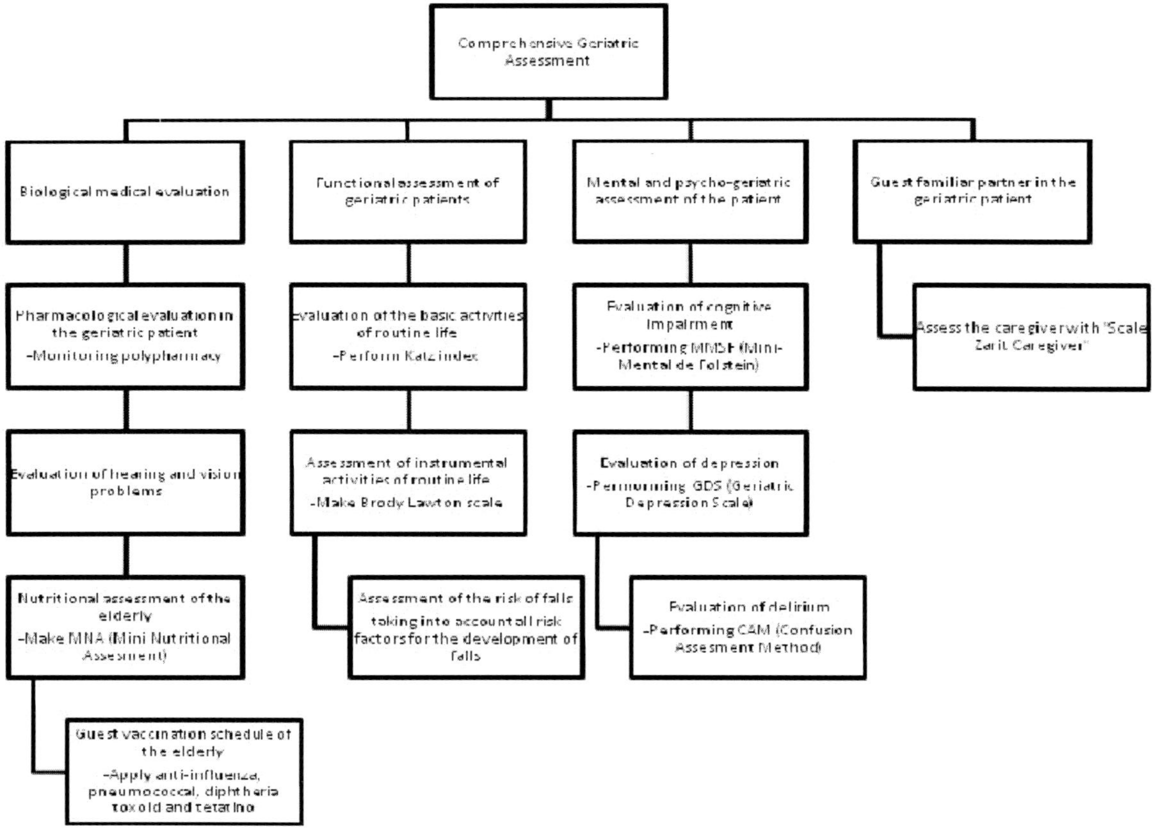

Figure 3. Comprehensive Geriatric Assessment in the elderly people.

Nonetheless, the purpose of this chapter is not to give a comprehensive description of each geriatric syndrome rather, it is to give a brief idea of the complexity of the issue as well as the complexity of assessing a geriatric patient. Figure 3 shows a diagram of the main aspects to be assessed which is drawn from data of Gerontological Comprehensive Geriatric Assessment in the elderly in our country [10].

SPECIFIC PATHOLOGIES BY ORGANS AND SYSTEMS IN THE ELDERLY PEOPLE

The elderly people as well as any other subject are prone to suffer some pathologies that may affect any organ or system, however, some diseases are seen in higher frequency in the elderly population. Table 2 shows the diseases most prevalent in older adults worldwide [1-3, 7, 11].

Table 2. Principal diseases that affect older people

Disease	Characteristics
Diseases of the sense organs	
Cataracts	Loss of transparency in the eye lens (crystalline) gives rise to visual impairment and which may progress to blindness.
Glaucoma	The optic nerve is damaged due to increased intraocular pressure. The vision is progressively reduced and may lead to blindness. This process usually begins in adulthood.
Hearing loss	Progressive decrease in hearing acuity. It is usually bilateral.
Central Nervous System Diseases	
Alzheimer's disease and other dementias	Neurodegenerative diseases characterized by loss of recent memory.
Parkinson´s disease	Slow and progressive degeneration of brain nerve cells leading to tremors, muscle stiffness, and mobility and balance difficulties

Disease	Characteristics
	Cardiovascular Diseases
Cerebral Vascular Disease	Provoked by partial or total occlusion of a brain blood vessel. The principal manifestations are: It causes symptoms such as weakness, loss of sensation in a body part, unilateral visual disturbance, Speech and comprehension difficulties and loss of balance or coordination.
Hypertension	It is an increase in systolic blood pressure above 140 mmHg and diastolic above 90 mmHg.
Ischemic Heart Disease	Refers to the partial or total occlusion of the coronary arteries which produces transient periods of ischemia and then myocardial necrosis.
	Gastrointestinal Diseases
Peptic-Ulcer Disease	Loss of substance of the digestive tract, causing ulcers in stomach and duodenum mainly.
Gastroesophageal Reflux Disease	It is a disease characterized by food regurgitation, chest pain. In severe cases it can progress to Barrett's esophagus, which is a precursor to esophageal adenocarcinoma.
	Metabolic Diseases
Diabetes Mellitus	The body does not respond to the action of insulin, causing a state of hyperglycemia and damage to the vessels and nerves. This disorder usually occurs in adulthood.
	Genitourinary diseases
Atrophic Vaginitis and Atrophic Urethritis	Characterized by thin vaginal walls and urethral tissues respectively producing pain during intercourse and burning sensation on urinating.
Bening Prostate Hyperplasia	Enlargement of the prostate gland that leads to urinary obstruction.
Prostate Cancer	Disproportionate growth of malignant cells in the prostate that gives rise to urinary obstruction, metastases and death.
Urinary Tract Infection	Colonization of bacteria in urine causing urinary symptoms.
	Musculoskeletal diseases
Osteoartrhitis	Degeneration of the cartilage lining the joints with resultant pain. It usually begins in adulthood.

Table 2. (Continued)

Disease	Characteristics
Miscellaneous	
Polypharmacy	Simultaneous use of 3 or more medical drugs with their underlying side effects.
Pressure Ulcers / Bedsores	The skin suffers an injury due to prolonged pressure that reduces blood flow to the affected area.
Periodontal Diseases	Term that refers to multiple alterations in the oral cavity, such as caries, periodontitis, edentulia among others.
Cancer in any organ in the body	Refers to an increased and uncontrolled growth of malignant cells in any organ. It can metastasize and cause death of the individual.

DISEASES BY ORGANS IN THE ELDERLY PEOPLE

Eye Diseases

Within the natural aging process there are certain ophthalmologic entities worth mentioning. Among these are the following:

Cataract

This is defined as a loss of transparency in the lens which conditions visual loss. Cataract is considered as the leading cause of reversible blindness worldwide. The risk factors in gerontological context are multifactorial. However, it is known that the main risk factor for suffering them is frequent exposure to UVB rays, and it is seen as a natural oxidation process of the lens. It commonly begins at the age of 60 years.

Treatment for this entity is exclusively surgical and postoperative pharmacologic management with steroids and ocular hypotensive drugs in some cases. Oral drugs used in this case may be prednisone and acetazolamide. The later may produce adverse effects like hypokalemia with serious secondary changes in elderly patients. For this reason, its use should be with care and only under prescription [12-14].

Glaucoma

It is defined as a loss of the fibers of ganglionic cells of the retina that form the optic nerve and are often prone to suffer elevated intraocular pressures. This pathology has multiple factors for their appearance and it is divided into different groups with open and closed angle glaucoma being the most frequents. This condition irreversibly affects the visual acuity and constitutes the leading cause of irreversible blindness worldwide.

Treatment of this disease is aimed at stopping the progression of visual loss, which is controlled by topical hypotensive medication but the use of carbonic anhydrase such as acetazolamide, to lower intraocular pressure, is prohibited in this age group [12, 15].

Hearing Diseases

The most common hearing impairment is presbycusis, which is the most frequent sensory disability in people of 65 years and above. It is a neurodegenerative disease that is commonly associated with aging and occurs earlier in men. The decrease in hearing acuity is attributed to the deterioration of the sensory cells and cochlear neurons which undoubtedly are non-regenerative cells. Clinically, it first affects the perception of high frequencies resulting in the loss of high frequency hearing. Hearing loss in older adults can lead to depression, social isolation, and loss of self-esteem [16]. Some environmental factors such as noise, chemicals, infections, lifestyle, drugs, mutations in mitochondrial DNA, metabolic diseases, diabetes and hypertension may contribute to the rapid deterioration of the disease [17]. The therapeutic approach is mainly hearing aids, however the knowledge and acceptance of the benefits of this therapy is still low. If hearing loss is excessive, surgical treatment as cochlear transplant is required. Apparently there is no drug therapy that could help or ameliorate the disease process [18].

Diseases of the Central Nervous System

Alzheimer's Disease (AD)

AD is considered the most common neurodegenerative disease in the elderly people. It is estimated that the disease affects 13 million Americans, and more than 24 million people worldwide. The projected estimate for the disease in 40-50 years is 81 million people. AD is characterized by progressive cognitive deficits and behavioral disturbances, accompanied by diffuse brain abnormalities. It is usually more prevalent in women [19].

Alzheimer´s disease is divided into 2 groups: Early AD (<60 years), considered as familial AD and characterized by mutations in APP gene (Amyloid Precursor Protein) and late onset or sporadic AD (> 60 years) which, is the most common presentation. The biggest risk factor for its development is the old age. People having a first-degree relative with dementia, have a higher risk with a probability of 10-30% of developing the disease when compared with the general population [20]. Apart from old age, other risk factors for developing AD are APOE genotype, female gender, high cholesterol, depression and head injury [20].

The typical manifestation of Alzheimer's disease is gradual and progressive loss of recent memory depicted in the patients by their inability or difficulty to remember conversations, dates, appointments and usually forget objects at home. Loss of memory leads to alterations in the patient's functional status. Another important feature of the patients is language dysfunction observed in up to 50% of the case manifested by "expressive aphasia," that is, difficulty in finding the words to use. When this disease progresses, it is common to see personality changes. In more severe stages, the patient may have confusion, dysphagia and repeated falls [19].

Currently, there is no study outlining the guidelines for a confirmatory diagnosis of AD in a living patient. Until date, the diagnosis is basically clinical, and the studies showing a definitive diagnosis have all been post-mortem where the pathological data include neuritic plaques (senile), amyloid angiopathy, neurofibrillary tangles and varying degree of microscopic cortical atrophy [21].

The management is usually multidisciplinary. The medical treatment is based on acetylcholinesterase inhibitors (rivastigmine, donepezil, galantamine). These drugs increase the levels of acetylcholine in neuronal synapses which increases cholinergic activity in affected brain regions. Cognition improvement has not been observed with the drug however, it slows the progression of cognitive impairment. The main side effects are nausea, anorexia, diarrhea and sleep [19-21].

Parkinson's Disease

Parkinson disease can occur at any age, but its peak of incidence is at 60 years of age. Parkinson disease is characterized by degeneration of the substantia nigra, and dopaminergic neurons, resulting in a deficiency of dopamine. It is also characterized by an increase in glial cells, and loss of neuromelanin of substantia nigra. The cause of this disease is still unknown [22, 24].

The main symptoms of Parkinson disease are: decreased facial expression, stooped posture, resting tremor (account currency), bradykinesia, and rigidity. These symptoms are caused by dopamine deficiency. The clinical diagnosis is made with the presence of tremor, rigidity and bradykinesias, responsive to levodopa. In the pathological study, paleness of the substantia nigra and locus ceruleus is found [24].

Treatment of the disease consists of three main categories: physical and mental health therapy, medication and surgery. So far, the best treatment is dopamine replacement drugs. The most potent among these drugs is levodopa, the immediate precursor of dopamine, usually administered with peripheral decarboxylase inhibitor to prevent the formation of dopamine in peripheral tissues.

Although**,** levodopa is the most effective drug, about 60% of the patients develop dyskinesia after five years of treatment, and patients under 60 are more likely to develop these problems before. Because of this, we recommend to start with other drugs such as amantadine, MAO inhibitors, anticholinergics and dopamine agonists [23].

Next in potency for the treatment of the disease symptoms are dopamine agonists like pergolide, bromocriptine and cabergoline. These drugs may induce fibrosis (valvulopathies, retroperitoneal, retroperitoneal and pleuropulmonar fibrosis).

Amantadine has multiple effects among which are antimuscarinic, activation of dopamine release from nerve terminals and blockage of dopamine entry at the nerve terminals. Dopaminergic action of amantidine helps to alleviate symptoms in approximately 2/3 of the patients [22, 23].

Stroke

It is considered that stroke is the 3rd leading cause of death in the United States as well as the main cause of disability. The incidence increases with age and approximately two-thirds of all strokes occur in people older than 65 years old [25].

Stroke is caused by a partial or complete occlusion of an intracranial artery or vein leading to a series of neurological deficits that serve as guides to locate the site of occlusion [25, 26].

Depending on their origin, strokes can be divided into two main groups: ischemic and hemorrhagic. Ischemic strokes are the most common type. It consists of approximately 80-90% of all the cases and can be thrombotic or embolic. The hemorrhagic type is usually more aggressive and represents approximately 20% of the cases of strokes. Within this group, we can identify two principal types: subarachnoid and intraparenchymal hemorrhages.

The main mechanisms by which occlusions of the intracranial arteries or veins occur are due to:

- Intrinsic condition of the vessel as atherosclerosis, vasculitis, and amyloid deposit.
- Vascular obstruction as cardiac embolism or the level of extracranial vessels (level of the internal carotid is more frequent).
- Cerebral hypoperfusion secondary to hypotension or blood viscosity.
- Rupture of an intracranial blood vessel.

The main risk factors for developing a stroke are: hypertension, diabetes, smoking, hypercholesterolemia, abnormal heart rhythm (atrial fibrillation, and acute myocardial infarction) [25, 26].

Because of the extent of this topic, we refer only to ischemic stroke which is subdivided into transient ischemic attack (TIT) and stroke. Transient ischemic attack (TIA) refers to the presence of a neurological deficit of less than 24 hours, while stroke is the presence of this condition for more than 24 hours. The later is usually secondary to decreased blood flow in a vascular territory. Table 3 shows the most affected vascular territories and its main clinical manifestations.

Table 3. Principal vascular territories affected by stroke and their clinical manifestations

Vascular Territory	Clinical Manifestations
Internal Carotid Artery	Unilateral amaurosis fugaz
Anterior Cerebral artery	Contralateral hemiparesis and hemihypoesthesia characterized by decreased spontaneous speech activity, grasp reflex and sucking. In some cases, there could be apraxia of gait.
Middle Cerebral Artery	It is the most affected artery. Contralateral hemiparesis and hemianopsia, Broca's or Wernicke's aphasia.
Posterior Cerebral Artery	Contralateral hemianopsia with respect to macular vision. There may be alexia and acalculia.

Diagnosis of stroke is done on the basis of the aforementioned clinical manifestations and on a simple cranial computerized tomography (CT) to differentiate hemorrhagic stroke from an ischemic one. Also, studies like electrocardiogram and blood count are necessary and facilitate the determination of the cause of stroke. Angio-tomography is usually done as a supporting study to the previous tests.

The objectives of medical treatment are to restore blood flow to the ischemic area which could be achieved by applying general measures as avoidance of rising temperature, hyperglycemia and sudden increase or drop in blood pressure. If the patient has less than 3 hours of onset of clinical manifestations, the attending physician should start with the administration of plasminogen activator factor (PAF). However, the administration should be done with care and individualized since the drug can lead to bleeding.

Drugs that are used as secondary prophylaxis administered alone or in combination with drugs such as diuretics, beta blockers, calcium antagonists, angiotensin converting enzyme (ACE) inhibitors, angiotensin receptor antagonists (ARA2) are mainly for the control of blood pressure. However, when they are combined with lipid control drugs as statins and antiplatelet therapy as ASA, clopidogrel, or anticoagulant therapy with warfarin, the possible pharmacological interactions that may arise among them should be born in mind [25, 26].

Cardiovascular Disease

Hypertension

Hypertension is one of the most prevalent diseases worldwide. It is a condition that occurs more frequently with increasing age and the prevalence is more in males than in females. It is defined as the elevation of systolic or diastolic blood pressure above 140 mmHg and 90 mmHg respectively [27, 28]. It is considered as one of the major risk factors for developing cardiovascular disease. Moreover, it is attributed to an increasing risk for kidney disease, atrial fibrillation, heart failure and stroke [27, 28].

Hypertension is classified as:

- Primary or essential hypertension characterized by multifactorial origin representing about 95% of patients with hypertension.
- Secondary hypertension resulting from a specific source with renal artery stenosis being the principal etiology.

In older adults, it is unusual to observe isolated elevated diastolic values, a condition that gave rise to the classification of systolic pressure into stages as:

- Stage 1: Systolic pressure between 140-159mmHg
- Stage 2 Systolic pressure ≥ 160mmHg

The elevation of blood pressure have various origins among which obesity, lack of exercise, insulin resistance, impaired-angiotensin-aldosterone system etc. can be highlighted [28, 29]. Table 4 shows the physiological changes in adulthood that contribute to increased blood pressure.

Due to the hidden nature or lack of manifested clinical signs, hypertension is considered as a "silent killer." Usually, when clinical manifestation appears, the life of the patient is already in danger. Chronic high blood pressure causes damage mainly at the level of retinal, renal, heart and brain vessels. The diagnosis is made by measuring blood pressure at rest on 3 different occasions with blood pressure (BP) greater than 140 / 90mmHg and discarding any secondary origin.

The goals of treatment are to maintain BP below 140 / 90mmHg. The treatment should begin with changes in lifestyle include avoidance of sedentary life and obesity. If the blood pressure does not decrease with these measures, drug therapy should be added. The main adverse effect of antihypertensive therapy is orthostatic hypotension [27-29].

The choice of drug for the control of blood pressure requires comprehensive review of the patient, considering other comorbidities. Table 5 shows the main advantages and disadvantages of the principal antihypertensive drugs.

Table 4. Physiological changes in adulthood that condition increased blood pressure

Arterial stiffness
Decrease in the sensitivity of the baroreceptors
Increased activity of the sympathetic nervous system
Decreased responsiveness of beta-adrenergic receptors
Endothelial dysfunction
Decreased sodium excretion capacity
Central obesity

Taken from: Hazzard's Geriatric Medicine and Gerontology 6e.

Table 5. Advantages and Disadvantages of antihypertensives in the elderly

Antihypertensive	Advantages	Disadvantages	Recomenmendation	Situations in which its use is not recommended or required monitoring
Diuretics: thiazide	Documented benefit in clinical trials -Produces Greater reduction in systolic and diastolic pressure -Improves bone mineral density -Low Cost	-Metabolic Alterations (hypokalemia) -Urinary frequency	Systolic hypertension	-Gout -Hyponatremia
Inhibitors of angiotensin converting enzyme (ACE)	-Absence of effects on CNS -Renal function preservation -Decreases proteinuria	-Hyperkalemia -Cough	-Heart failure -Diabetes Mellitus	-Renal failure -Renal artery stenosis.
Beta adrenergic antagonists	It is not recommended as monotherapy	- Can increase peripheral vascular resistance -oxidative metabolic alterations -Effects on CNS	Myocardial postinfarction	- COPD (Chronic Obstructive Pulmonary Disease) -Peripheral Vascular Disease -Block heart -DM type 2 -Hyperlipidemia
Antagonists, alpha-adrenergic receptors	Improves urinary symptoms in BPH (benign prostatic hyperplasia)	It increases the frequency of hospitalizations for heart failure when used as monotherapy	Prostatism	Left ventricular disfunction

Taken, edited and translated from Hazzard's Geriatric Medicine and Gerontology 6e.

Ischemic Heart Disease

Ischemic heart disease has a wide spectrum of clinical manifestations:

- Stable angina
- Acute coronary syndromes
    - Unstable angina
    - Acute myocardial infarction without ST segment elevation
    - Acute myocardial infarction with ST-segment elevation

This type of disease is more common in men of 50 years old and above. Women in pre-menopausic age have a lesser risk of suffering the disease due to estrogenic effect. However, post-menopausic women have the same risk of ischemic heart disease. The main risk factors predisposing this disease is hypertension, diabetes mellitus, atherosclerosis, obesity, smoking, alcoholism, sedentary lifestyle [30, 31].

Within the pathophysiology is endothelial damage leading to formation of atherosclerotic plaques whose calcification may result in the breakage of the blood vessel. Consequently, this activates the coagulation system causing thrombotic blood clots that occlude the coronary arteries [30, 31].

The typical manifestations of coronary arterial disease are oppressive type of chest pain that radiates to left shoulder and jaw, with a feeling of impending doom, accompanied by nausea, vomiting, sweating and incontinence. Besides patients refer to dyspnea, abdominal pain, confusion, and discomfort which can be misinterpreted as some other pathology [30-32]. Usually, death after coronary heart disease occurs in people over 65 years old [30].

Diagnosis requires evaluation of 3 parameters:

- Clinical manifestations that are compatible with ischemic heart disease.
- Electrocardiographic data showing the damage or ischemia or necrosis of cardiac muscle.
- Elevated cardiac troponin with its respective enzyme curve.

Based on these 3 parameters physicians could reach a definitive diagnosis of coronary arterial disease in some of its variants.

The treatment of acute coronary syndrome is based on the acronym "MONA" meaning Morphine-Nitroglycerin-Oxygen-Aspirin. In addition, depending on the patient's hemodynamic status, other drugs such as pravastatin and beta-blockers, can be included Depending on the time of evolution, thrombolysis may result from drugs whose main side effect is bleeding. However, when the effect of these drugs is not favorable, coronary revascularization may be performed. Revascularization procedure is however not within the scope of the purpose of this chapter [32].

Gastrointestinal Diseases

Peptic Ulcer Disease

This disease is characterized by secretion of a substance into the protective mucous lining of the digestive tract that is damaging to this lining thereby predisposing the tract muscles to lesions which eventually lead to its perforation. Ulcers are classified as gastric or duodenal depending on their location.

The general incidence of this disease has decreased in the last 100 years, although in older adults the prevalence still persists [33]. The main complications of ulcers in their order of frequency are bleeding, perforation and obstruction [34].

It is known that the main risk factors for developing ulcers are the intake of NSAIDs and active *H. pylori* infection. Because older adults tend to self-medicate with NSAID, they are more susceptible to development ulcers. Approximately 20% of these ulcers in older adults are not associated with *H. pylori* infection or NSAID intake [33], about 25% of duodenal ulcers and 40% of gastric are associated with the intake of NSAIDs or aspirin respectively [33].

The typical clinical manifestations are pain, epigastric burning, which can improve with food (duodenal) or not (stomach), and can be accompanied by nausea, vomiting and anorexia. However, in older adults these manifestations are not so clear, hence endoscopic study is recommended in all patients with new abdominal symptoms [33]. *H. pylori* detection studies have to be carried out. In case it is positive, it needs to be eradicated using triple scheme based on double dose of proton-pump inhibitor + amoxicillin + clarithromycin. It has been shown that this scheme in older adults for a week is well tolerated and very effective [33]. The doses of NSAIDs should be reduced in those patients whose underlying disease requires chronic intake of the drug. The main drug used for this disease is the proton-pump inhibitor [33-34].

Gastroesophageal Reflux Disease (GERD)

This is a common condition in the extreme of life. Its principal symptom is regurgitation of food. It may be accompanied by chest pain, burning sensation in the chest, chronic or nocturnal cough, laryngitis, and probably pneumonia. Differential diagnosis of the chest pain is necessary to discard acute myocardial infarction.

The pathophysiology of reflux is due to transient relaxations of the lower esophageal sphincter. Other common alterations in elderly are excessive saliva secretion, delayed gastric emptying, and less resistant gastric mucous [33]. Certain drugs such as theophylline, calcium channel blockers, benzodiazepines, dopaminergics, tricyclic antidepressants and anticholinergics increase the risk of GERD. These drugs are often used in geriatrics.

When older people do not present the typical manifestations of the disease, it is recommendable to carry out an endoscopic study to determine the degree of esophagitis or some other etiology of the disease [33]. The major complications of GERD are erosive esophagitis, Barrett's esophagus and esophageal adenocarcinoma in less than 1% [35].

Metabolic Diseases

Diabetes Mellitus Type 2 (DM2)

Type 2 diabetes mellitus is a metabolic disorder characterized by an alteration in the metabolism of glucose, lipids and proteins, causing generalized vascular damage. It is a disease that has increased in incidence and prevalence in young people. In the United States of America, more than 50% of people with diabetes are over 60 years [36]. According to the National Factor Sheet 2011, diabetes affects 8.3% of Americans of all ages, 11.3% of adults aged older than 20 years [37].

Type 2 diabetes mellitus is frequently seen in obese, sedentary and hypertensive patients. Common laboratory finding is asymptomatic hyperglycemia i.e., high blood sugar. The classic symptoms of diabetes are polydipsia, polyuria and polyphagia that may be accompanied by weight loss [36]. It is important to mention that diabetes mellitus has a wide spectra of manifestations, which depend on the age of the patient. Table 6 shows these differences.

Table 6. Manifestation of diabetes mellitus according age of patients

Metabolic Abnormality	Young patient	Elderly patient
Increase of osmolarity	Polydipsia	Dehydration, confusion, decreased visual acuity
Glucosuria	Polyuria	Urinary incontinence
Catabolic state	Polyphagia due to lack of insuline	Weight loss, Anorexia

The main complications of this disease can be classified in acute and chronic. Acute complications include diabetic ketoacidosis, hyperosmolarity and hypoglycemia. These complications are more common in patients with type 1 diabetes, or patients with poor therapeutic control. Chronic complications are most important because these are the main causes of mortality and morbidity. These complications include diabetic retinopathy, which can lead to blindness, diabetic nephropathy leading to end-stage renal disease and peripheral neuropathy, which is clinically known clinically as "diabetic foot" and constitutes the leading cause of infections and amputations [39]. DM2 diagnoses are based on the criteria of ADA (American Diabetes Association) Table 7 [36, 38].

Table 7. Diagnostic Criteria for Diabetes Mellitus according to ADA

1. Glycated Hemoglobin A1c (HbA1c) ≥ 6.5%
2. Glucosa in more than 126 mg/dL in fasting (no food intake for at least 8 hours before the test)
3. Glucose levels ≥200 after performing glucose tolerance curve with 75g oral glucose
4. Random plasma ≥200 with the classic symptoms of diabetes: polydipsia, polyuria, polyphagia.

* The presence of at least one of the following criteria is required.

The treatment should be integral and not only to decrease the level of glucose or maintain it at normal level but also to manage all the ensuing cardiovascular risk factors such as hypertension, high levels of cholesterol, hyperlipidemia etc.

According to ADA, glycemic control can be assessed by HbA1c ≤ 7, but should be individualized for each patient. The glycemic levels may be treated according to the type of diabetes with insulin or with hypoglycemic drugs such as sulfonylureas, biguanides, tiazolinedionas, nateglinidas, although the strict surveillance of these drugs is very important to evaluate the main side effect provoked by situations of hypoglycemia [36].

Genitourinary Diseases

Benign Prostatic Hypertrophy (BPH)

BPH is a disease that often occurs with increasing age. The diagnosis is based on histological analysis. The prevalence of BPH in men aged 50-69 years is 25% and over 80% in men aged 70-79 years [40].

BPH is a pathology that is characterized by increase in the size of the prostate manifested by symptoms of urinary obstruction regardless of changes in the organ size, cell proliferation or cellular dysfunction.

Among the main risk factors leading to the development of BPH are obesity, race (more common in black people), diabetes, excessive alcohol consumption, and physical inactivity [40].

The main clinical manifestations are related with lower urinary tract symptoms such as urinary hesitancy, urine stream weakness, post-void dribbling, and incomplete bladder emptying.

To carry out an accurate diagnosis of BPH requires, in occasions, the biopsy of the gland, where glandular and fibromuscular growth is reported. Since biopsy is an invasive and traumatic study, it is not the first choice. Some physicians use the IPSS test (International Prostate Symptom Rating) as a supporting diagnosis. The IPSS test is a questionnaire consisting of seven questions that evaluate the major symptoms of the disease, and the feeling of the patient in terms of life quality with the symptoms. Based on the result, a treatment plan is designed to tackle the problem.

The principal drugs of use for the treatment of BPH are alpha-adrenergic blockers that ameliorate the urinary symptoms and inhibitors of 5-alpha-reductase to inhibit glandular growth.

In case of mild symptoms (score <7IPSS), "watchful waiting" can be applied with changes in the lifestyle together with the administration of an alpha-adrenergic blocker such as tamsulosin. However, the adverse effects as headache, orthostatic hypotension (that provoke falls in older adults), retrograde ejaculation and dizziness should be carefully monitored. In addition to the above is dutasteride, an inhibitor of 5-alpha-reductase, whose effects on prostate growth is reached at 6 months. The main side effects of this drug are impotence, decreased libido and gynecomastia, effects that lead to cut down the duration of treatment [40, 41].

Urinary Tract Infection (UTI)

UTI refers to bacterial colonization in the bladder which is usually a sterile cavity. This disease is more prevalent in older adults. Most of the time, it is asymptomatic. Symptomatic situations are usually associated with serious morbidity problems [42]. In women, it is more common in older people and mainly manifested as asymptomatic bacteriuria. The main etiological agents are *Escherichia coli, Klebsiella pneumoniae, Staphylococcus saprophyticus, Enterococcus faecalis, group B Streptococcus (GBS), Proteus mirabilis, Pseudomonas aeruginosa, Staphylococcus aureus and Candida* [43]. The infection has a broad spectrum of clinical manifestations that go from acute uncomplicated urinary infection, no obstructive pyelonephritis, infection of complicated urinary tract, asymptomatic bacteriuria, acute prostatitis to chronic bacterial prostatitis. Lower UTI usually provokes dysuria, increased urinary frequency, urinary urgency, suprapubic pain and incontinence [42, 43].

The presence of fever, flank pain and lower urinary tract symptoms are important symptoms leading to the suspicion of acute pyelonephritis unless otherwise proved. In the presence of the clinical manifestations, it is pertinent to carry out urine analysis in search of clinical manifestations like leukocytes, hematuria, nitrites +, presence of bacteria, leukocyte esterase+ as a diagnostic support. A definitive diagnosis is reached through urine culture with a count of 100,000 CFU (CFU = colony forming units) with "midstream" sample. Moreover, the study permits the establishment of the etiologic agent and microbial sensitivity. Imaging studies are reserved for cases in which complications are suspected. The treatment for UTI as cystitis and pyelonephritis is based on TMP / SMX, nitrofurantoin, ciprofloxacin, or fluoroquinolones for 10 days [42, 43].

Miscellaneous

Polypharmacy is defined as the use of multiple medications by a patient. The minimum number of medications required to apply the term of “polypharmacy” is variable and ranges from 5 to 10 drugs [44] including those that are not prescribed by a doctor such as herbs, tea, vitamin supplements and others.

Because elderly patients have a higher prevalence of the diseases, this group of people is more likely to have multiple concurrent medications.

The main problem of polypharmacy is that the simultaneous use of multiple medications increases the risk of adverse effects regardless of patient´s age [45] and such use may lead to physiological changes due mainly to the long duration of drugs in the body. Additional risk of polypharmacy is the possible interaction between them and intoxication at this stage of life [46]. It is important to mention that certain drugs increase the risk of falls in older adults and this usually results in hip fracture. This is the reason why falls on geriatric syndrome provoke high morbidity and mortality. Moreover, polypharmacy can influence "prescription cascade" [47].

Adverse Drug Reactions (ADR)

ADR refers to any damage that occurs after to drug administration and this includes harmful responses, errors in drug administration, and any other circumstance that could cause harm. There are several factors in the elderly that contribute to increase the development of drug-related problems. These factors are fragility, coexisting medical conditions, multiple prescriptions and self-medication custom [48].

Budnitz et al., found that in the period between 2007 and 2009 in the United States, 99.628 people over 65 years old were admitted in the emergency unit due to adverse effects of drugs and that 2/3 of these were related dosages [47]. In other patients with chronic diseases, the risk of drug interactions increases for the multiple drugs required to control their disease.

Table 8. Drugs that could lead to a waterfall prescription

Initial Pharmacological Therapy	Adverse Event	Subsequent Pharmacological Therapy
Antipsychotics	Extrapyramidal signs and symptoms	Anti-Parkinson therapy
Cholinesterase inhibitors	Urinary incontinence	Incontinence Treatment
Thiazide diuretics	Hyperuricemia	Gout treatment
NSAIDs	Increased blood pressure	Antihypertensive therapy

Taken from Rochon PA, Gurwitz JH. BMJ 1997.

Waterfall Prescription

This is a term that refers to the administration of one new drug to treat any new symptoms, when in fact the "new symptoms" are caused by an adverse effect of the drug of base [48]. This phenomenon increases the risk of developing new adverse effects due to the new drug. Older adults with increased risk of this phenomenon are those with chronic degenerative diseases. Table 8 shows the principal drugs that can lead to a waterfall prescription.

Cancer

Cancer is defined as an uncontrolled growth of malignant cells that could spread from one tissue or organ to another. It is a disease that can develop in any part of the body [49, 50]. Age is the biggest risk factor for developing cancer. Cancer cells must have certain characteristics to be considered as such i.e., increased growth rate, invasion of adjacent tissues and the ability to metastasize [51].

The name given to any cancer is based on the tissue of origin, for example, those deriving from epithelial tissue are called carcinomas, and those from hematopoietic cells, leukemia or lymphomas.

The cellular and molecular changes that occur in a cancer cell are very complex issue. Therefore, it is important to know that the vast majority of cancers are due to many genetic abnormalities that contribute to loss of control of cell growth, increased capacity to invade and survive outside the original tissue by angiogenesis.

The World Health Organization (WHO) refers to cancer as the leading cause of death worldwide and reported 8.2 million deaths in 2012. It is the second leading cause of death in the United States after heart disease. The main types of cancer generally seen worldwide are lung, liver, gastric, colorectal, breast and esophageal cancers [50]. Development of cancer is multifactorial (Figure 4).

The main modifiable risk factors for the development of cancer are consumption of excessive alcohol, smoking, high-fat containing and low fiber diets as well as sedentary lifestyle. However, certain viruses as HPV (Human Papillomavirus), HBV (Hepatitis B Virus) and HCV (Hepatitis C Virus) are capable of causing cancer [49, 50].

Cancer is an inherent disease in adulthood. This is probably due to the accumulation of cell mutations, exposure to various environmental factors and an unhealthy life style for several years. So, it is necessary that older people implement screening studies to detect the disease at its early stage for timely treat in order to have opportunity of better survival and good life quality.

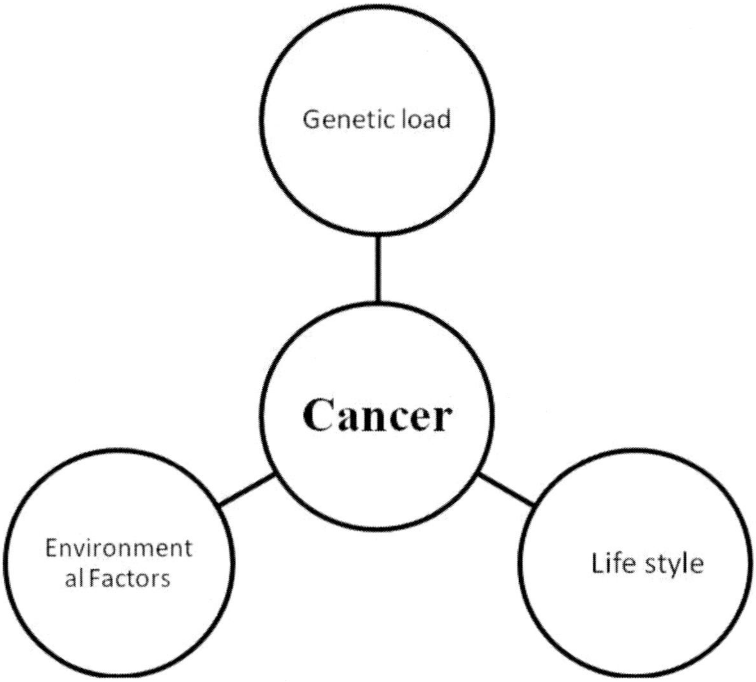

Figure 4. Factors that influence the development of cancer.

CONCLUSION

The study of elderly people is very complex. The objective of this chapter is to explore the principal diseases that affect the elderly people and to highlight that in spite of their increasing comorbidities, physicians should always try to prescribe only the essential drugs in small doses and enlighten them on the risk of polypharmacy and the "prescription cascade" as well as having in mind that an integral evaluation of geriatric population is of paramount importance. The following chapters of the book will address and analyze the pharmacokinetic profiles of elderly people as instruments for developing better drug schemes that would maintain adequate drug levels necessary for their therapies with an eye to avoiding adverse drug effects or therapeutic fails.

REFERENCES

[1] Miller R.A. (2009). Chapter 1. Biology of Aging and Longevity. In Halter J.B., Ouslander J.G., Tinetti M.E., Studenski S, High K.P., Asthana S (Eds), *Hazzard's Geriatric Medicine and Gerontology,* 6e.

[2] Davies, A.M, "Ageing and healt in the 21st century: an overview. *Proceedings of a WHO Symposium. Kobe,* 10-13 November, 1998.

[3] WHO: Ageing. Available in: http://www.who.int/topics/ageing/es/.

[4] José, J., & García, G. (2010). Health and disease in older adults. 239–248.

[5] Health Ministry. Ageing Care. First Edition, Mexico City, Mexico. Guralnik J.M., Ferrucci L (2009). Chapter 5. Demography and Epidemiology. In Halter J.B., Ouslander J.G., Tinetti M.E., Studenski S, High K.P., Asthana S (Eds), *Hazzard's Geriatric Medicine and Gerontology*, 6e.

[6] Lozano Ascencia, Frenk Mora et al. The burden of disease in the elderly. Mexico 1994, Public Health of Mexico. 38: 6, 1996

[7] Carlson Charlotte, Merel E. Susan et al. Geriatric Syndromes and Geriatric Assessment for the Generalist. *Med Clin N Am* 99 (2015) 263–279.

[8] Liu D, Walter LC. Prevention and Health Promotion. In: Williams BA, Chang A, Ahalt C, Chen H, Conant R, Landefeld C, Ritchie C, Yukawa M. eds. *Current Diagnosis and Treatment: Geriatrics,* Second Edition. New York, NY: McGraw-Hill; 2014.

[9] Guide for Clinic Practice. Geriatric Gerontological Health Checking. IMSS 491-11. Available in: http://www.cenetec.salud.gob.mx/descargas /gpc/CatalogoMaestro/491_GPC_valoracixn_geronto-geriatrica/IMSS-491-11-GER.

[10] Kuchel G.A. (2009). Chapter 51. Aging and Homeostatic regulation. In Halter J.B., Ouslander J.G., Tinetti M.E., Studenski S, High K.P., Asthana S (Eds), *Hazzard's Geriatric Medicine and Gerontology,* 6e.

[11] Whiteside M (2014). Managing Vision Impariments in Older Adults. In Williams B.A, Chang A, Ahalt C, Chen H, Conant R, Landefeld C, (Eds), *Current Diagnosis and Treatment: Geriatrics,* Second Edition.

[12] Yanoff, M. and Duker, J. S. (2014). Basic Science of the Lens. *Ophthalmology* (Fourth Edition). Elsevier Ltd. http://doi.org/10.1016/B978-0-323-04332-8.00057-3.

[13] Bron, A. (1192). The ageing eye. In G. J. Evan and F.T Williams (Eds.) *Oxford textbook of geriatric medicine* (pp557-574).

[14] Yanoff, M. and Duker, J. S. (2014). Epidemiology and mechanism of Glaucoma. *Elsevier* Ltd. http://doi.org/10.1016/B978-0-323-04332-8. 00057-3
[15] Kim TS, Chung JW. Evaluation of age-related hearing loss. *Korean J Audiol.* 2013 Sep;17(2):50-3. doi: 10.7874/kja.2013.17.2.50. Epub 2013 Sep 24.
[16] Kee YK. Pathophysiology of age-related hearing loss (peripheral and central). *Korean J Audiol.* 2013 Sep;17(2):45-9. doi: 10.7874/kja.2013. 17.2.45. Epub 2013 Sep 24.
[17] Sha S, Talaska A.E., Schacht J (2009). Chapter 44. Age-Related Changes in the Auditory System. In Halter J.B., Ouslander J.G., Tinetti M.E., Studenski S, High K.P., Asthana S (Eds), *Hazzard's Geriatric Medicine and Gerontology,* 6e.
[18] Carlsson C.M., Gleason C.E., Puglielli L, Asthana S (2009). Chapter 65. Dementia Including Alzheimer's Disease. In Halter J.B., Ouslander J.G., Tinetti M.E., Studenski S, High K.P., Asthana S (Eds), *Hazzard's Geriatric Medicine and Gerontology*, 6e.
[19] Van Duijn, Clayton D, et al. Familial aggregation of Alzheimer's disease and related disorders: a collaborative re-analysis of case-control studies. Risk Factors Research Group. *Int J Epidemiol.* 1991;20 Suppl 2:S13.
[20] Matthew (2010). Chapter 28: Central Nervous System. In Robbins L, Cotran KA, Aster F. Structural and Functional Pathology. 8ed.
[21] Fahn S (2009). Chapter 66. Parkinson's Disease and Related Disorders. In Halter J.B., Ouslander J.G., Tinetti M.E., Studenski S, High K.P., Asthana S (Eds), *Hazzard's Geriatric Medicine and Gerontology*, 6e.
[22] Connolly BS, Lang AE. Pharmacological treatment of Parkinson disease: a review. *JAMA.* 2014 Apr;311(16):1670-83.
[23] Matthew (2010). Chapter 28: Central Nervous System. In Robbins L, Cotran KA, Aster F. Structural and Functional Pathology. 8ed.
[24] Smith W.S., Johnston S, Hemphill J, III (2015). Cerebrovascular Diseases. In Kasper D, Fauci A, Hauser S, Longo D, Jameson J, Loscalzo J (Eds), *Harrison's Principles of Internal Medicine,* 19e.
[25] CTO Neurology and Neurosurgery Manual 7th edition. McGraw Hill. Interamericana.
[26] Supiano M.A. (2009). Chapter 81. Hypertension. In Halter J.B., Ouslander J.G., Tinetti M.E., Studenski S, High K.P., Asthana S (Eds), *Hazzard's Geriatric Medicine and Gerontology*, 6e.

[27] Syed Q, Messinger-Rapport B (2014). Hypertension. In Williams B.A., Chang A, Ahalt C, Chen H, Conant R, Landefeld C, Ritchie C, Yukawa M (Eds), Current Diagnosis and Treatment: Geriatrics, Second Edition.

[28] Arterial Hypertension. Guide for Clinic Practice. Available in: http://www.cenetec.salud.gob.mx/descargas/gpc/CatalogoMaestro/238_IMSS_09.

[29] Peterson E.D., Gharacholou S.M. (2009). Chapter 76. Coronary Heart Disease. In Halter J.B., Ouslander J.G., Tinetti M.E., Studenski S, High K.P., Asthana S (Eds), *Hazzard's Geriatric Medicine and Gerontology,* 6e.

[30] Dhruva S, Cheitlin M (2014). Coronary Disease. In Williams B.A., Chang A, Ahalt C, Chen H, Conant R, Landefeld C, Ritchie C, Yukawa M (Eds), *Current Diagnosis and Treatment: Geriatrics*, Second Edition.

[31] Ibrahim, A. W., Riddell, T. C. and Devireddy, C. M. (2014). Acute myocardial infarction. *Critical Care Clinics,* 30(3), 341–364.

[32] Pilotto A, Franceschi M (2009). Chapter 91. Upper Gastrointestinal Disorders. In Halter J.B., Ouslander J.G., Tinetti M.E., Studenski S, High K.P., Asthana S (Eds), *Hazzard's Geriatric Medicine and Gerontology,* 6e.

[33] Kitagawa Y, Dempsey D.T. (2014). Stomach. In Brunicardi F, Andersen D.K., Billiar T.R., Dunn D.L., Hunter J.G., Matthews J.B., Pollock R.E. (Eds), *Schwartz's Principles of Surgery,* 10e.

[34] Jobe B.A., Hunter J. G., Watson D. I. (2014). Esophagus and Diaphragmatic Hernia. In Brunicardi F, Andersen D. K., Billiar. T.R., Dunn D.L., Hunter J.G., (Eds), *Schawartz´s Principles of Surgery*, 10e.

[35] [36] Powers A.C. (2012). Chapter 344. Diabetes Mellitus. In Longo D.L., Fauci A.S., Kasper D.L., Hauser S.L., Jameson J, Loscalzo J (Eds), *Harrison's Principles of Internal Medicine,* 18e.

[36] U.S Department of Healt and Human Services, Centers for Disease Control and Prevention, 2011. National Diabetes fact sheet: national estimates and general information in diabetes and prediabetes in the United States, 2011. Available at http://www.cdc.gov/diabetes/pubs/pdf/ndfs_2011.pdf. Accessed January 5, 2014.

[37] [Guideline] Diagnosis and classification of diabetes mellitus. *Diabetes Care*. Jan 2012;35 Suppl 1:S11-63.

[38] Pollock, F., &Funk, D.C. (2013). Acute Diabetes Management. *AACN Advanced Critical Care,* 24(3), 312-324.

[39] Sarma V. Aruna; Wei. T. John. Bening Prostatic Hyperplasia and Lower Urinary Tract Symptoms. *N. Engl J. Med* 367:3 July 19, 2012.

[40] Chao S, Chippendale R (2014). Benign Prostatic Hyperplasia and Prostate Cancer. In Williams B.A., Chang A, Ahalt C, Chen H, Conant R, Landefeld C, Ritchie C, Yukawa M (Eds), *Current Diagnosis and Treatment: Geriatrics,* Second Edition.

[41] Nicolle L.E. (2009). Chapter 127. Urinary Tract Infections. In Halter J.B., Ouslander J.G., Tinetti M.E., Studenski S, High K.P., Asthana S (Eds), *Hazzard's Geriatric Medicine and Gerontology*, 6e.

[42] Flores-Mireles AL, Walker JN, et al. Urinary tract infections: epidemiology, mechanisms of infection and treatment options. *Nature Reviews Microbiology.* Volume 13. Mayo 2015.

[43] Ferner RE, Aronson JK. Communicating information about drug safety. *BMJ.* 2006;333(7559):143.

[44] Field TS, Gurwitz JH, Avorn J et al. Risk factors for adverse drug events among nursing home residents. *Arch Intern Med.* 2001;161(13):1629.

[45] Weng MC, Tsai CF, et al. The impact of number of drugs prescribed on the risk of potentially inappropriate medication among outpatient older adults with chronic diseases. *QJM.* 2013 Nov;106(11):1009-15. Epub 2013 Jul 8.

[46] Budnitz DS, Lovegrove MC, et al. Emergency hospitalizations for adverse drug events in older Americans. *N Engl J Med.* 2011;365(21):2002.

[47] Rochon PA, Gurwitz JH. Optimising drug treatment for elderly people: the prescribing cascade. *BMJ.* 1997;315(7115):1096.

[48] WHO- Cancer. Available in: http://www.who.int/mediacentre/factsheets /fs297/es/.

[49] National Cancer Leadership Congress 2014. Disponible en: http://www.uicc.org/national-cancer-leadership-congress-2014.

[50] Thomas P. (2010). Chapter 7. Neoplasms. Robbins and Cotran. Structural and Functional Pathology, 8 ed. Elsevier.

In: Optimization of Drug Prescribing in Elderly ISBN: 978-1-63484-879-4
Editors: Juárez O. H. and Lares A. I.

Chapter 3

EFFECT OF AGE ON THE PHARMACOKINETIC OF DRUGS IN ELDERLY

Hugo Juárez Olguín[1,*], David Calderón Guzmán[2] and Stephanie R. Pérez Saldaña[3]

[1]Laboratorio de Farmacología, Instituto Nacional de Pediatría, Mexico City, Mexico and Departamento de Farmacología, Facultad de Medicina, Universidad Nacional Autónoma de Mexico, Mexico

[2]Laboratorio de Neurociencias, Instituto Nacional de Pediatría, Mexico City, Mexico

[3]Departamento de Farmacología, Facultad de Medicina, Universidad Nacional Autónoma de Mexico, Mexico City, Mexico

ABSTRACT

Elderly people are characterized by degenerative changes in the structure and function of organs and tissues. The most important changes in the body composition are related to water, protein and fat balance. These changes modify the volume of distribution. A downward tendency

---

* Corresponding author: Hugo Juárez Olguín, Laboratorio de Farmacología, Instituto Nacional de Pediatría. Avenida Imán # 1, 3er piso, Col Cuicuilco, CP 04530, Mexico D.F, Mexico, e-mail: juarezol@yahoo.com.

of the volume of distribution increases the initial peak plasma concentration and the site of action. Physiological changes over the years are generally produced in a predictable manner. Individual characteristics and variabilities play an important role in the speed or rate of aging. This speed or rate for different specific physiological functions regularly and linearly declines although, there are other functions that relatively remain unchanged and only decline at the end of life or when a disease develops. Knowledge of the physiology of aging reveals the importance of rational drug use in the elderly and permits its practice in this group of the population. This work reviews the physiologic changes that affect the pharmacokinetic profiles on the basis of which a better therapeutic scheme could be developed to handle the complicated health problems of the elderly population with an eye to adapting the drug to the patient and not viceversa.

INTRODUCTION

Aging is a phenomenon marked not only by physical and structural degenerative changes but also by functional changes in the organs and tissues. The speed of these degenerative changes varies depending on individual characteristics. Hence, two patients of 75 years under the same pathological conditions may react very differently to the injection of the same dose of a drug with the elimination time being totally different. This means that an individual can be functionally older than another of the same chronological age. The process occurs in various parts. Body composition changes with an increase in the lipid fraction and a loss of skeletal mass. Also, this is affected by a decrease in body water and protein, especially albumin. Deep understanding of pathophysiological and pharmacological principles in relation to the changes occurring in these factors in this age group is essential for proper pharmacological management [1].

Physiological changes over the years are generally produced in a predictable manner and these depend on individual characteristics and variabilities, that is, the speed or rate of aging for specific physiological functions regularly or linearly declines. However, other functions remain relatively unchanged and decline only at the end of life or when a disease develops.

The structural and functional degenerative changes in organs and tissues due to aging virtually occur at subcellular and tissue levels and some organs are clearly defined to suffer age-related functional alterations [2]. Although, the function of these organs can be kept at a minimum, they can still be maintained at an appropriate level and this often requires daily administration of medications.

In different studies, it was found that age is correlated with two mortality peaks, at the early and final stages of life. It was observed that mortality increases gradually with age until 85 years old and from then on, this increase becomes accelerated. Hence mortality in elderly patients is directly proportional to the age. The effect of age on people older than 80 years supposed to be increased morbidity and mortality, but contrary to expectations, the percentage of complications (death) is constant. This means that there should be some other factors, beside age, that are responsible for death in elderly people.

For medical practices, the most important changes in the organs are those related with cardiovascular system, liver and kidney [3]. Muscle is an important tissue that is affected by aging. At 30 years old, 15% of the muscle tissue is replaced by fat while at 65 years the rate increases to 30% and this can increase to 40% in women. The coexistence of multiple diseases provides a competitive morbidity and mortality risk. Different pathophysiological changes are due to reduced functional reserve which increases the problem and simulates pathological event which in fact is inexistent.

PHARMACOKINETIC CHANGES

The most important change in body composition is the water-protein-fat relationship. This change modifies the volume of distribution (Vd) which affects the plasma concentration. Reduced volume of distribution increases the initial peak plasma concentration and the site of action. The volume of distribution can also be affected by changes in cardiovascular system. Decreased cardiac output at rest and prolongation of circulation time lead to a slower onset of action, mainly in the brain and generally less compensatory response [4]. The variation in the pharmacodynamics of drugs also explains the increased sensitivity to certain drugs or the poor response of others. It is also necessary to emphasize that a patient consuming numerous drugs for control of his or her diseases is required to have current knowledge of the possible drug interactions and most importantly, the altered physiology of the elderly [5]. Aging is a property of living matter and therefore an irreversible physiological process. As humans grow older, the cells and tissues become less efficient and less able to replace damaged tissues.

A feature of this group of patients is the marked variability of physiological parameters which makes the task of distinguishing the processes of aging difficult from the diseases associated with aging. In order to provide a secure and predictable therapy, it is necessary to take this into account. We should bear in mind that biological age, which varies from one organism to another, is more important than chronological age [6].

Knowledge of the physiology of aging could give way to the rational use of drugs in the elderly people. The major physiopathological reasons leading to different magnitude of responses to drugs are as follows:

- A lower volume of distribution.
- Reduced number of proteins that bind to drugs.
- Increase in the relative concentration of the receivers.
- Decreased ability of the liver in the detoxification processes.
- Lesser ability of the kidney to eliminate drugs and their metabolites.

All these physiological problems bring about abnormal responses to drugs and to other substances used for purposes other than therapeutic agents or adjuvants. Basically these changes directly alter two biological processes:

- The volume of distribution (Vd).
- Metabolism and excretion.

While indirectly, they affect

- Plasma elimination half-life.

VARIATIONS IN THE DISTRIBUTION OF DRUGS

The volume of human body decreases as people get older. This reduces the volume in which drugs are distributed and increases the plasma concentration of the same. A knowledge of this concept is important for drug-dose adjustment and prevention against the high incidence of adverse effects and drug interactions common in the elderly patients. Plasma albumin levels decrease with age consequently, there are less drug-binding sites which in turn increase the amount of free drug in the plasma. The increase in diffusion gradient would require greater and faster transfer site and cellular action.

Changes in tissue processes such as relative composition; the amount of water, lipids and proteins as well as the rate of tissue irrigation are all factors of variation in drug response. Another important factor influencing drug response variation is the body's response to the effects of drugs. Reduced, cardiac reserve or decreased cerebral blood flow predisposes to an exaggerated slow response to intravenous and inhalational agents [7]. A comprehensive knowledge of all the physiological or pathophysiological changes that occur in elderly patients would allow physicians to predict the differences in the magnitude of the effect of drugs. To anticipate the complications, it is pertinent to remember that due to decreased plasma protein, muscle mass and increased body fat, there are pharmacologically pharmacodynamic and kinetic changes of drugs. BMR decreases with age by 1% after 30 years and hence, drugs are metabolized more slowly.

Drug Metabolism

Variations in drug metabolism differ considerably in each individual. In the elderly, there is reduced blood flow as liver mass gets reduced. This loss of tissue by the liver gives rise to a declination in its functions. Proteins, mainly albumin, are produced by the liver. Therefore a decrease in serum albumin will bring about reduced binding sites for drugs. This alteration in the protein is one of the most important pharmacokinetic variants because reduction in proteins permits a greater fraction of free drug to enter the cells and bind to receptors.

The ability to metabolize drugs in the liver appears to decrease with age. Clinical studies suggest that certain drugs are metabolized more slowly. The most significant changes occur in phase I and some of these changes are due to decreased hepatic blood flow and altered volume of distribution.

Effects on Protein Binding

Primary binding sites of plasma proteins are albumin and alpha1-acid glycoprotein. Albumin decreases with age and this alters the bioavailability of certain drugs that bind to proteins and increases the alpha1-acid glycoprotein. The effects of these changes therefore depend on which of the two proteins is the primary binding site and the relative impact is on the clearance of the free fraction and volume of distribution. For example, diazepam binds primarily to albumin therefore, in the elderly patients, the free fraction is increased. This means that the requirement of this drug by elderly people should be less otherwise they should have greater amount of free drug (activated drug) in plasma. Another example is lidocaine which primarily binds to alpha 1-acid glycoprotein. Hence in elderly patients, the free fraction of lidocaine is decreased and the clearance is reduced [8]. Many drugs are extensively metabolized by the liver. Without significant contribution of extrahepatic sources, the hepatic clearance depends on three factors:

- Union of drug proteins
- Liver flow
- Extrinsic metabolic capacity of the liver for drug disposal.

The pharmacokinetics of drugs change with age. As age increases, there is a delay in the elimination half-life and an increase in the volume of distribution. For instance, diazepam has an average life of 20 hours in people aged 20 years. This means that in older people, the average life of the drug is higher. Transpolated to elderly people, the average life of diazepam is equal in hours to their age. In the case of Lorazepam, the pharmacokinetic and the metabolic pathway are only slightly altered by age. These kinetic changes are due to changes in protein binding and distribution of fat and water in the body.

All patients who have decreased cardiac output have less liver flow and thus slow metabolism and prolonged drug action. It is therefore necessary that intervals of drug consumption be based on real duration of drug action according to ages and not just repeating doses at a set intervals.

Glomerular filtration rate decreases from 45 to 50% between 20 and 90 years. In elderly, there is diminished capacity to concentrate urine and excrete hydrogen ions. As people get older, the ability of the kidney to excrete endogenous creatinine reduces [9]. This index is used to correlate the actual dosage of those drugs that are excreted by this route.

Receptor Binding

Most drugs used by the elderly bind to receptors. Many studies have shown a decrease in some hormones and drugs, as well as a variation in affinity for the same. An example of this is the cardiac beta receptor. A lower response to isoproterenol and increased adverse effects of β-blockers are observed. On the other hand, there is a group of receptors that relatively increase with age. In fact, what relatively decreases are the cell components as water which explains the increase in the number of receptors per unit area.

In the elderly, there is a generalized depletion of neurotransmitters like dopamine, norepinephrine, tyrosine, serotonin, and a simultaneous increase in enzymes as monoamine oxidase and catechol-O-methyltransferase activity, which are essential for the metabolism of neurotransmitters [10]. As a result, Parkinson and Alzheimer diseases reflect specific neurotransmitter deficiency and are most commonly seen in the elderly pathologies. The global cerebral blood flow (CBF) falls in proportion to the reduction of brain mass; any decrease in CBF is a consequence not a cause of brain atrophy [11].

Changes in Liver Function

Liver size decreases markedly with age. Approximately 40-50% of the adult liver tissue may regress 80 years and hepatic blood flow is proportionally reduced. However, there is a qualitative change in small hepatocellular function. The loss of well perfused liver tissue appears to play an important role in reducing the clearance of drugs related to age. The rate of hepatic clearance of drugs that require hepatic biotransformation is reduced especially those that follow a 1st mechanism step. Furthermore, hepatic synthesis of plasma cholinesterase and albumin is also deficient and this would lead to an altered pharmacokinetics of some drugs [12].

Variations of Renal Function

Renal blood flow is inversely related to age. The renal clearance is decreased in elderly patients even when creatinine is normal. The combination of these changes produces a gradual decline in glomerular filtration. As a result, the elderly patient is vulnerable to fluid overload and the cumulative effect of drugs that rely on renal clearance. The average time of renal elimination of certain drugs that are eliminated by this pathway and its metabolites is prolonged in the elderly, especially in those with preexisting renal insufficiency.

Despite the marked changes in renal functional reserve, serum creatinine concentrations usually remain within normal limits, since the decrease in skeletal muscle mass generates a progressively lower burden of creatinine. Decreased creatinine clearance obviously increases the concentrations and determines a delay in excretion of drugs that are eliminated by the kidney.

RENAL SYSTEM, DRUG AND ELECTROLYTE

Bilateral loss of renal tissue is approximately 30% at 80 years when compared with a young adult of 30 years. More than a third of the glomeruli and their associated structures is changed. The total renal flow decreases by 50%, a decrease of 10% every 10 years from early adulthood. Increasing age leads to atrophy of the kidney and compromises renal vasculature. The reduction of functioning glomeruli alters glomerular filtration efficiency. A deterioration in its function leads to retention of sodium and concentration of urine.

The ability to concentrate urine decreases with age, especially after fluid deprivation. It also impairs the ability to conserve sodium, making this age group susceptible to hyponatremia. Although older people release high concentrations of antidiuretic hormone in response to the load of hypertonic saline, water retention is less efficient than that seen in young adults, probably due to a decreased response of target organs to this hormone [13].

It should be remembered that digitalis is eliminated by the kidney and this can accumulate to toxic level if the function of the kidney is insufficient [14]. Moreover, antibiotics like aminoglycosides are also eliminated by the kidneys and their accumulation can empower high doses of muscle relaxants.

Another physiological function affected by the age is adrenergic response. The adrenergic responses also vary with age. Vasoconstrictor response to stress produced by cold, position changes, hypovolemia, etc., is decreased as people get older [15]. These alterations in vasomotor reactions to heat stress are only one of the causes of the relative inability of the elderly to deal with hypothermia.

The elderly people are more susceptible to delirium awakening as a result of different physical illnesses, stress, intoxication and drugs that are frequently used, even at therapeutic doses. Etiological factors are hypoxic (particularly anticholinergics, benzodiazepines and tricyclic) alcohol abuse, depression, dementia, metabolic disorders and drug interactions [16].

It is therefore advisable to avoid "polypharmacy" in the elderly since postoperative delirium is shown to be related to the number of prescribed medications.

Opiates also suffer significant pharmacodynamic and pharmacogenetic changes. Decrease in proteins increases the free fraction of opiates and decreases the volume of distribution. This means that more of these drugs can get faster to the central nervous system, [17] where there is a higher relative number of receptors for it and thus the action is more intense and the side effects such as cardiovascular and respiratory depression are more prolonged [18].

DRUG INTERACTIONS

The drugs taken by patients are usually prescribed by the physicians. The physician prescribing drugs should therefore have an excellent knowledge of the pharmacodynamics and pharmacokinetics of the drugs as well as their toxic side effects and their potentials to interact with each other [19]. Drug interactions affects the intensity of the response of the drugs involved. The end result may be an increase or decrease or even the cancellation of therapeutic effects. As elderly people are prone to concurrent polypharmacy for being fraught with different pathologies, the possibility of drug interaction is high. Some of these possible drug interactions are highlighted here.

Drugs used by cardiologist such as beta-blockers act on the calcium pump to depress or strengthen it. Inhalational agents block the entrance of calcium to heart cells, smooth muscle and skeletal tissues. Anesthetic agents act on endoplasmic reticulum and inhibit calcium transport activity and consequently sodium-calcium pump.

Drugs blocking slow calcium channels have inotropic effect by decreasing the contractions of the cardiac muscles as well as vasodilatation. Halothane decreases AV conduction at the node level and the enhancement of this effect could favor the onset of arrhythmias.

Abrupt withdrawal of beta-blocking drugs produces undesirable effects as tachycardia, severe hypertension, arrhythmias, and dangerous signs among others [20]. In the same manner, abrupt suppression of antiparkinson drugs such as levodopa produces neuroleptic malignant-like syndrome, including elevated body temperature and muscle stiffness.

CONCLUSION

Advances in the knowledge of aging physiology are recently gaining momentum in favor of improving the conditions and prolonging the life of elderly people. These studies have allowed the development of new concepts in pharmacology, separating the concepts of the effect of aging per se from the consequences of inter-current diseases of the elderly. From the third decade of life, aging causes progressive atrophy, fibrosis and loss of elasticity in virtually all tissues.

In the absence of disease, organ function remains adequate to meet the baseline requirements and even moderate demands. Aging causes a series of changes that alter the body's response to drugs. However, aging by itself, does not produce a disease state (old age), but the changes accompanying it which are part of a natural process could be faster or slower depending on the individual. However, chronological age produces a state of "dysfunction" which can advance to testable physiological dysfunctions.

As a group, seniors are prone to a higher risk of morbidity and mortality compared with younger subjects due to their high susceptibility to incidences of inter-current diseases that significantly lower their functional reserves and the maximum capacity of all their organ systems which predispose them to chronic intake of medication. It is important to reiterate that administration of drugs in this group of patients must take into considerations not only the chronological age dysfunctions but also the accompanying physiological dysfunctions in order to adapted drug prescriptions to the patient and not the patient to the drug.

REFERENCES

[1] Ginsberg G, Hattis D, Russ A, Sonawane B. Pharmacokinetic and pharmacodynamic factors that can affect sensitivity to neurotoxic sequelae in elderly individuals. *Environ Health Perspect.* 2005 Sep;113:1243-9.

[2] Beynon CM. Drug use and ageing: older people do take drugs! *Age Ageing* 2008, 22.

[3] Falck P, Asberg A, Byberg KT, Bremer S, Bergan S, Reubsaet JL, Midtvedt K. Reduced elimination of cyclosporine A in elderly (>65 years) kidney transplant recipients. *Transplantation.* 2008;86:1379-83.

[4] Gidal BE. Drug absorption in the elderly: biopharmaceutical considerations for the antiepileptic drugs. *Epilepsy Res.* 2006, 68 Suppl 1:S65-9.

[5] Haider SI, Johnell K, Weitoft GR, Thorslund M, Fastbom J. The Influence of Educational Level on Polypharmacy and Inappropriate Drug Use: A Register-Based Study of More Than 600,000 Older People. *J Am Geriatr Soc.* 2008, 14.

[6] Metlay JP. Medication comprehension and safety in older adults. *LDIIssue Brief.* 2008;14:1-4.

[7] Bellia V, Battaglia S, Matera MG, Cazzola M. The use of bronchodilators in the treatment of airway obstruction in elderly patients. *Pulm Pharmacol Ther.* 2006; 19:311-9.

[8] Pautex S, Vogt-Ferrier N. Management of chronic pain in older persons. *Rev Med Suisse.* 2006;2:1629-30

[9] Conil JM, Georges B, Lavit M, Seguin T, Tack I, Samii K, Chabanon G, Houin G, Saivin S. Pharmacokinetics of ceftazidime and cefepime in burn patients: the importance of age and creatinine clearance. *Int J ClinPharmacol Ther.* 2007; 45:529-38.

[10] Arlt S, Lindner R, Rösler A, von Renteln-Kruse W. Adherence to medication in patients with dementia: predictors and strategies for improvement. *Drugs Aging* 2008;25:1033-47.

[11] Allain H, Bentué-Ferrer D, Polard E, Akwa Y, Patat A. Postural instability and consequent falls and hip fractures associated with use of hypnotics in the elderly: a comparative review. *Drugs Aging.* 2005;22:749-65.

[12] Staatz CE, Tett SE. Pharmacokinetic considerations relating to tacrolimus dosing in the elderly. *Drugs Aging.* 2005;22:541-57.

[13] Staskin DR. Overactive bladder in the elderly: a guide to pharmacological management. *Drugs Aging.* 2005;22:1013-28.

[14] Barni S, Cabiddu M, Petrelli F. Toxicity of targeted therapies in elderly patients. *Expert Rev Anticancer Ther.* 2008, 8:1965-1976.

[15] Cassidy N, Lee SK, Donegan CF, Tracey JA. Poisoning in older adults: the experience of the national poisons information centre. *Ir Med J.* 2008;101:268-70.

[16] Howland RH. Risks and benefits of antipsychotic drugs in elderly patients with dementia. *J Psychosoc Nurs Ment Health Serv.* 2008;46:19-23.

[17] Hilleret H, Falconnet C, Le Saint L, Perrenoud JJ, Michel JP, Vogt-Ferrier N. Prescribing psychotropic drugs to patients aged 80 and over. *Rev Med Suisse*. 2008; 4(178):2405-8, 2410-1.

[18] Mangoni AA. Cardiovascular drug therapy in elderly patients: specific age-related pharmacokinetic, pharmacodynamic and therapeutic considerations. *Drugs Aging*. 2005;22:913-41.

[19] Perucca E, Berlowitz D, Birnbaum A, Cloyd JC, Garrard J, Hanlon JT, Levy RH, Pugh MJ. Pharmacological and clinical aspects of antiepileptic drug use in the elderly. *Epilepsy Res*. 2006; 68 Suppl 1:S49-63.

[20] Tsuyuki RT, McLean DL, McAlister FA. Management of hypertension in elderly long-term care residents. *Can J Cardiol*. 2008, 24:912-4.

In: Optimization of Drug Prescribing in Elderly ISBN: 978-1-63484-879-4
Editors: Juárez O. H. and Lares A. I. © 2016 Nova Science Publishers, Inc.

Chapter 4

USEFUL OF THE PHARMACOKINETIC STUDIES AS A BASE FOR THE ESTABLISHMENT OF THERAPEUTIC SCHEDULES

Radames Alemón Medina**, Juan Luis Chávez Pacheco and Gabriela Pérez Guillé

Laboratorio de Farmacología, Instituto Nacional de Pediatría, Mexico City, Mexico

ABSTRACT

Pharmacokinetic knowledge sets the principles and the bases for designing or modifying either the loading or maintenance dose of a treatment scheme, and the interval of administration of the drug. The establishment of a rational dosification scheme should take into consideration essential aspects as biological and physiopathological characteristics of the patient, the therapeutic range established and the pharmacokinetic of the patient himself. However, it is practically impossible to know the pharmacokinetic of the patient. Therefore, in the face of this impossibility, the therapeutic decision should be based on the knowledge on literature reports on pharmacokinetic parameters carried

* Corresponding autor: Radames Alemón Medina, Laboratorio de Farmacología, Instituto Nacional de Pediatría, Avenida Imán # 1, 3er piso, Col Cuicuilco, CP 04530, Mexico D.F, Mexico. E-mail: ranapez@hotmail.com.

out in patients with similar or likely biological and physiopathological characteristics as the patient under study.

In the same way, all those biological, genetic, physiological, physiopathological and pharmacogenetic/pharmacogenomic factors that could modify the treatment response as well as the dosification scheme should be considered. It is important to point out that from the pharmacokinetic knowledge the following questions could be satisfactorily answered:

1. What data are necessary to be used in designing a treatment scheme?
2. What are the essential pharmacokinetic parameters to get the loading and maintenance doses?
3. What are the biological, physiological and/or physiopathological factors that odify the pharmacokinetic parameters and their meaning?

The details of these concepts are described in this chapter.

INTRODUCTION

Pharmacokinetic studies provide the opportunity to learn from a quantitative point of view, the way in which the body of a person interacts with a drug administered to achieve a pharmacological response, and which is excreted by the different elimination mechanisms.

When making measurements of plasma levels of a drug administered either as a single dose or in multiple applications, and considering the changes that these concentrations undergo over the time, drug movement dynamics in the body can be understood. So, the determination or identification of the kinetics of each of the phenomena involved in the dynamics can be carried out based on the frequency of taking blood samples. These kinetic phenomena are: the kinetics of absorption, distribution (including major organs such as the brain), elimination and/or excretion.

Pharmacokinetic applied to the clinic is focused on accurate patient care and facilitates knowledge that would effectively contribute to the care of the sick. The development of this discipline should be of great interest to all professionals involved in healthcare.

DEFINITIONS AND FUNCTIONS OF CLINICAL PHARMACOKINETICS

Clinical pharmacokinetics is a discipline of Health Sciences, which is related to the application of pharmacokinetic principles to ensure safe and effective therapeutic management of any patient taking into consideration his/her individual characteristics. Its functions include [1]:

1. Designing Dose Regimens at the Beginning of Therapeutic Management

Establishment of an appropriate treatment regimen demands a consideration of the drug dose aspects, administration intervals, route of administration and pharmaceutical form. Unfortunately, these pharmacokinetic information is generally available in the literature and could be obtained from the patient himself when we take the trouble to make the pharmacokinetic study [2-3]. It is important to consider all the characteristics of the patient that may influence the pharmacokinetic behavior and consequently the therapeutic success. Among such characteristics are: age, sex, body weight or body surface area, race or other indicators of possible pharmacogenetic influences [4-5]. The later could be determined by genotypification of the gene polymorphisms that regulate drug metabolizing enzymes as is the case of cytochrome P450 (CYP450) enzyme complex that participate not only in response to treatment but also in its interindividual variability, for instance tamoxifen [6-8]. Moreover, it is important to consider the state of disease and its pathophysiological changes, kidney function, hematocrit, albumin, urinary pH, and the concomitant use of other drugs that can determine drug interactions.

2. Optimizing Therapeutic Management

If the therapeutic success is not achieved, it is important to know the aspects mentioned in point 1, and to review the patient's medication history from the point of view of individual pharmacokinetic analysis, and reset or redesign a new regimen based on this. Strategically, this is the "Therapeutic Drug Monitoring" [9-10], which directly or indirectly assesses clinical response to drug using plasma or other biological fluid concentrations of the drug in question. Moreover, it is important to check the quality of clinical records and the methods used in carrying out the drug monitoring. For example, is it based on clinical changes or on certain biochemical parameters?

3. Evaluation of Drug Therapy in Special Cases or in Drugs that Have a High Risk of Intoxication or Therapeutic Failure

This refers to patients with liver and/or renal damage, critically or seriously ill patients, people with nutritional disorders, patients with peritoneal dialysis and patients with acute drug intoxication. These classes of patients definitely require meticulous pharmacokinetic study for a better adjustment of the therapeutic regimen [11].

4. Retrospective Evaluation of Therapeutic Management

In order to detect errors that may have occurred in the management, distribution, preparation and/or administration of the treatment regimen, an assessment of how the above processes took place has to be conducted. This could be done during clinical visit, in hospital clinical sessions and post-mortem pathologic discussions.

5. Pharmacokinetic Database

It is useful to carry out pharmacokinetic studies in individuals of different ages, sex, race, nutritional status, health status, pathophysiological condition, as well as the use of multiple drugs in patients with various diseases in order to create data base of individuals under different biological and pathological conditions with different medications for consultations by physicians and those unable to perform pharmacokinetic studies due to technological limitations. The availability of a data base would provide elements for the therapeutic management of patients with pharmacokinetic criteria. The creation of a data base that contemplates physic-chemical and pharmacokinetic properties of drugs would be an invaluable source of knowledge to the physicians and would notably improve their understanding of the relationship between physic-chemical characteristics and disposition of the drug. It is pertinent to point out that timely pharmacokinetic studies would surely help to improve the efficacy and safety of drugs [12-13].

6. Pharmacokinetic Diagnosis

Treatment failure is not surprising in the clinical field and the observation of unusual or pronounced pharmacological responses to drug adverse effects is something very frequent. Well-targeted and properly conducted pharmacokinetic studies by a qualified professional should lead to the detection and identification of possible causes of treatment failure. Such possible causes could be bioavailability problems; errors in the prescription and in the drug; as a consequence of high prevalence of chronic degenerative disease as in the elderly people that require multiple drugs; drug interactions; failure by the patient; unusual behaviors in the kinetics of distribution and elimination or certain pharmacodynamic effects include alterations in the interaction with receptors on the sites of action [14-16].

7. Research in the Field of Pharmacokinetics

The activities to be developed in this field should focus on identifying and controlling the causal factors influencing the dynamics for biodegradation and excretion of a drug in the diseased patient. An example is the existence of interactions between genes and drugs that could have an impact on the functions of some organs. This could be exemplified in elderly adults where the prescription of some high risk drugs is based on comorbidity and functional state of the patient [17-18]. When a pharmacokinetic study is performed, it is necessary to control all the variables which can alter each of the biological pharmacokinetic parameter depending on individual characteristics, target organs, changes in body composition and other simultaneous controls [19-20].

It is extremely important to consider all these points of investigations, which could be laborious and complicated due to the level of specialization of the human resources and materials needed to implement them anywhere in practical and easily applicable way. In Mexico, not all hospitals have the resources to undertake these studies, however, it is, at least, expected that highly specialized hospitals dedicated to this type of researches should use their experience and acquired knowledge in pharmacokinetic field to conduct studies that would generate useful information to be applied in any level of healthcare regardless of having or not technological resources. The essential thing is to achieve a change of attitude in the therapeutic management of patients based on avoiding therapeutic failures and obtaining optimum therapeutic benefits by applying pharmacokinetic criteria originating from highly specialized research centers.

8. Educational Activities

In addition to what is proposed in the above, it is extremely important to guide healthcare personnels through educational activities based on pharmacokinetic knowledge so as to ensure that medicines are used safely and effectively [21].

References

[1] Levy G., *An orientation to clinical pharmacokinetics.* In Clinical Pharmacokinetics: A Symposium, Levy, G., Ed., American Pharmacology Association. Washington, D.C., 1974, 1-9.

[2] Mehvar R. Pharmacokinetic- based design and modification of dosage regimen. *Am J Pharm Educ* 1998; 62:189-95.

[3] Holford NHG, and Sheiner LB. Kinetics of pharmacologic response. *Pharmacol Ther* 1982; 16(2): 143-66.

[4] Franconi F, Campesi I. Sex and gender Influences on pharmacological response: an overview. *Expert Rev Clin Pharmacol* 2014; 7(4)469-85.

[5] Koch HJ, Rascha C. Anthropometic data and acetylsalycilic acid pharmacokinetics. *Int J Clin Pharmacol Ther* 2002; 40(1):30-4.

[6] Franconi F, Camposi I. Pharmacogenomics, pharmacokinetics and pharmacodynamics: interaction with biological differences between men and women. *Br J Clin Pharmacol* 2014; 171(3):580-94.

[7] De VriesSchultink AH, Zwart W, Linn SC, Beijnen JH, Huitema AD. Effects of pharmacogenetics on pharmacokinetics and pharmacodynamics of tamoxifen. *Clin Pharmacokinet* 2015; 54(8):797-810.

[8] Samer CF, Lorenzini KI, Rollason V, Daali Y, Desmeules JA. Aplications of CYP450 testing in the clinical setting. *Mol Diagn Ther* 2013; 17(3): 165-84.

[9] Ghiculescu RA. Therapeutic drug monitoring: which drug, why, when and how to do it. *Aust Prescr* 2008; 31:42-44.

[10] Reid CM. The role of clinical registries in monitoring drug safety and efficacy. *Heart Lung Circ.* 2015 Jul 6. pii:S1443-9506(15)00392-3. doi: 10.1016/j.hlc.2015.04.184. [Epub ahead of print].

[11] Hvidberg EF. Why do we need pharmacokinetics studies? *Am J Obstet Gynecol* 1990: 163 (1 Pt2):316-18.

[12] Obach RS, Lombardo F, Waters NJ, Trend analysis of a database of intravenous pharmacokinetic parameters in human for 670 drug compounds. *Drug MetabDispos.* 2008 Jul; 36(7):1385-405.

[13] Walker DK. The use of parmacokinetic and pharmacodynamics data in the assessment of the drug safety in early drug development. *Br J Clin Pharmacol* 2004; 58(6)601-08.

[14] Opondo D, Eslami S, Visscher S, de Rooij SE, Verheij R, Korevaar JC, Abu-Hanna A. Inappropiateness of medication prescriptions to elderly patients in the primary care setting: a systematic review. *PLoS One*; 2012; 7(8):e43617. doi:1371/journal.pone.0043617. Epub 2012 Aug 22.

[15] Cahir C, Fahey T, Teeling M, Teljeur C, Feely J, Bennett K. Potentially inappropriate prescribing and cost outcomes for older people. *Br J Clin Pharmacol* 2010; 69(5):543-52.

[16] Gupta M, Awarwai M. Understanding medication errors in the elderly. *N Z Med J.* 2013; 126(1385):62-70.

[17] Li J, Kim S, Sha X, Wiegand R, Wu J, LoRusso P. Complex disease-gene-, and drug-drug interactions: impacts of renal function, CYP2D6 phenotype, and OCT2 activity on veliparib pharmacokinetics. *Clin Cancer Res* 2014; 20(15):3931-44.

[18] John V, Mashru S, Lichtman S. Pharmacological factors influencing anticancer drug selection in the elderly. *Drugs Aging* 2003; 20(10):737-59.

[19] Benet LZ, editor: *The effect of Disease States on Drug Pharmacokinetics.* Academy of Pharmaceutical Sciences. American Pharmaceutical Association, Washington, D.C. 1976.

[20] Ritchel WA, editor: *Physiological and Pathologic Factors Influencing Drug Response*. In: Handbook of Basic Pharmacokinetics. Hamilton, IL 62341: Drug Intelligence Publications, Inc.: 1980. Chapter 30.

[21] Huges GJ, Cassagnol M, Wu W, Howland MA, Sym D, El-Chaar GM, Smith CJ. Modification of a pharmacokinetics course design to improve student performance. *Am J Pharm Educ* 2014; 78(5):93.doi 10.5688/ajpe 78593.

In: Optimization of Drug Prescribing in Elderly ISBN: 978-1-63484-879-4
Editors: Juárez O. H. and Lares A. I. © 2016 Nova Science Publishers, Inc.

Chapter 5

MEANING OF PHARMACOKINETIC PARAMETERS

***Hugo Juárez Olguín*[1,*]*, Stephanie R. Pérez Saldaña*[2] *and Ismael Lares Asseff*[3]**

[1]Laboratorio de Farmacología, Instituto Nacional de Pediatría, Mexico City, Mexico and Departamento de Farmacología, Facultad de Medicina, Universidad Nacional Autónoma de México, México D.F., México

[2]Departamento de Farmacología, Facultad de Medicina, Universidad Nacional Autónoma de México, México City, México

[3]Centro Interdisciplinario de Investigacion para el Desarrollo Integral Regional (CIIDIR), Instituto Politécnico Nacional, Durango, México

ABSTRACT

A pharmacokinetic parameter is an essential data, a variable or a factor to evaluate changes which certain situation or substance can undergo when subjected to certain condition. Drugs when administered undergoes a series of certain changes governed by a kinetic reaction process measured by their velocity to be liberated, absorbed, distributed, metabolized or excreted (LADME System).

* Corresponding author: Hugo Juárez Olguín: Laboratorio de Farmacología, Instituto Nacional de Pediatría. Avenida Imán # 1, 3er piso, Col Cuicuilco, CP 04530, Mexico D.F, Mexico. E-mail: juarezol@yahoo.com.

From each of these kinetic processes of velocity, a measurement of the functional capacity as well as the participating enzymatic system in each of the processes is obtained. The values gotten in these measurements are considered as markers of the functional capacities to eliminate a foreign body/substance as food, drugs, poison, environmental pollutants or any xenobiotic substance from the body. The obtained pharmacokinetic parameters corresponding to each of the kinetic process of absorption, distribution, metabolism and excretion are individual measurements unique for every person and every one of them is subject to intra and interindividual variability in line with the pharmacogenetics and biological processes as well as physical activities and environmental factors in which the person is exposed. This gives rise to the importance of individualization or personalization of a treatment regimen taking into account the characteristics of every patient.

Presently, the establishment of a treatment regimen ought to be based on preventive pharmacogenetics diagnoses and optimization that are achieved from a pharmacokinetic knowledge of each patient and with orientation towards personalized pharmacotherapy.

INTRODUCTION

The biological half-life ($t_{½el}$), the apparent volume of distribution (Vd), clearance (Cl) and the bioavailability of drugs are pharmacokinetic concepts that are used to describe and predict the time course of the plasma concentrations of a drug depending on the dose and frequency of administration. Moreover, they are also used to characterize the patient's individuality, including the effects of the disease according to kinetics of absorption, distribution, metabolism and excretion [1].

Applying these principles to the clinic would permit the introduction of the pharmacokinetics in medical practice, which would help to the understanding and optimization of the therapeutic management of patients. Only through understanding the dynamic behavior of the body on the drug, can we answer the following questions arising when carrying out a therapeutic plan:

- How many?
- How?
- At what time and how often should a drug be administered to achieve sustained therapeutic levels?

- What settings should the dosing regimen for patients with kidney failure be?
- Can a drug be administered only once instead of three times a day?
- When can blood samples be obtained to monitor drug concentrations?
- What is the probability that a patient has a drug intoxication, and the probability of therapeutic success?
- How many days of treatment are required to obtain the maximum therapeutic effect of a treatment regimen?
- How are we going to identify and handle a patient who behaves as slow or as fast eliminator of a drug?

The application of pharmacokinetic principles allows us to evaluate and improve medication therapy, with the purpose of helping the doctor with the design of dosing regimens that would achieve plasma concentrations and the desired therapeutic response. The response of the body to a drug administered involves taking into account a multiplicity of interacting variables such as age, sex, nutritional status, habits like smoking or drinking alcoholic beverages and disease states. Although, plasma concentration achieved is not definitely the end of the treatment but the aim is to reach a level within a therapeutic range that would prevent the occurrence of acute attacks of certain diseases such as cardiac arrhythmias, asthma or seizures. However, monitoring the drug concentrations will never replace the clinical judgment of the doctor but would serve to enrich well-being of the patient.

SYSTEMIC BIOAVAILABILITY

The amount of drug that reaches the general circulation is considered as the systemic bioavailability of the drug [2, 3]. When a drug is administered intravenously, it is considered to have absolute bioavailability which means that it has complete systemic bioavailability, although this cannot happen when it comes to prodrugs that require some processing which sometimes may be incomplete.

When a drug in its various presentations – tablets, capsules suspension or suppositories, etc. is orally administered, the active substance which includes various forms of excipients has to be released. Once the active ingredient is released, it undergoes enzymatic chemical changes that is absorbable in the stomach and small intestine and hence goes to the liver and finally emptied into the circulation. The amount of drug that passes through the liver to blood circulation for distribution in the body is considered as the bioavailable quantity of the drug [4].

The bioavailable quantity of a drug can be measured by comparing the area under the plasma concentration curve of the drug versus time after oral administration with the bioavailability of the same dose administered intravenously. The proportion of both curves indicates the bioavailable amount [5].

Biological Half-Life

For drugs that are orally administered, the concept expresses the time required for the concentration of the drug to decrease by 50% after absorption and distribution and determines the duration of the drug effect and its persistence in the body. In most cases, it is independent of dose, concentration, or the route of administration. The biological half-life can be obtained directly from the slope corresponding to the linear phase after absorption and distribution by the plasma concentration versus time on a semi-logarithmic scale [6].

Apparent Volume of Distribution

The apparent volume of distribution does not represent a real space. It comprises of the volume in which a drug is distributed, which can be as small as the plasma volume distribution, that is 5% of total volume, or it may reach several hundred liters, depending on the amount of drug that binds to plasma proteins and tissue proteins. It denotes the apparent volume necessary to contain the entire amount of a drug, if the drug in the entire body were in the same concentration as in the plasma. The apparent volume of distribution expresses the relation between the amount of drug in the body and the plasma concentration after the drug has been absorbed and distributed [7].

Renal Clearance

This concept may be defined as the volume of blood that is completely cleared of a drug or any other substance administered in the body per unit time. It is equal to the rate of excretion divided by the average concentration of the substance in plasma [8, 9]. Renal clearance of a drug in a person with normal renal function may vary from patient to patient, and from time to time, depending on urinary pH, urinary flow rate, drug binding to proteins and blood flow to the kidney. The clearance also describes how efficiently a body eliminates a drug, so it is a constant of proportionality that relates the rate with the volume of distribution [10].

Total Clearance

It is the rate of clearance of a drug by the body as a whole divided by the average concentration. Therefore, it is the sum of the partial clearances of a drug by different organs and tissues [10].

Factors Influencing Treatment Response

The pharmacokinetic parameters could be affected by biological and physiopathological factors such as age, sex, body weight, nutritional condition, genetic and environmental factors as well as circadian rhythms all of which determine changes in chronopharmacokinetic and response to treatment [11].

References

[1] Brüggman J. Clinical Importance of pharmacokinetic parameter. *Hospital Pharmacy Europe Issue 36 January/February 2008.*

[2] WA Ritchel, editor: Bioavailability and Bioequivalence. In: *Handbook of Basic Pharmacokinetics*. Hamilton, IL 62341: Drug Intelligence Publications, Inc.: 1980. Chapter 31 p 382-409.

[3] Schumacher GE. Interpretation of bioavailability data by practitioners. *J Clin Pharmacol.* 1976; 16(10 Pt 2):554-9.

[4] Canada AT. The importance of bioavailability to the pharmacist. *Int J Clin Pharmacol Biopharm*. 1975;11(4):346-8.

[5] Toutain PL and Bousquet-Melou. Bioavailability and its assessment. *J Vet Pharmacol Ther*. 2004;27:455-66.

[6] WA Ritchel, editor: Determination of Rate Constants. In: *Handbook of Basic Pharmacokinetics*. Hamilton, IL 62341: Drug Intelligence Publications, Inc.: 1980. Chapter 17. P 208-218. *Am J Hosp Pharm*. 1983 Oct;40(10):1637-41.

[7] Bauer LA. Primer on clinical pharmacokinetics. *Am J Hosp Pharm* 1983;40 (10): 1637-41.

[8] Gibaldi M, Levy. Pharmacokinetics in clinical practice. I. Concepts. *JAMA*. 1976 26;235(17):1864-7.

[9] Gibaldi M, Levy G. Pharmacokinetics in clinical practice. 2. Applications. *JAMA*. 1976 May 3; 235(18):1987-92.

[10] Paxton JW. Elementary pharmacokinetics in clinical practice 2: Basic concepts of drug pharmacokinetics. *N Z Med J*. 1981; 94(695):342-5.

[11] W Ritchel, editor: Physiological and Pathologic Factors Influencing Drug Response. In: *Handbook of Basic Pharmacokinetics*. Hamilton, IL 62341: Drug Intelligence Publications, Inc.: 1980. Chapter 27.

In: Optimization of Drug Prescribing in Elderly ISBN: 978-1-63484-879-4
Editors: Juárez O. H. and Lares A. I.

Chapter 6

RELEVANCE OF THE PHARMACOKINETIC APPLIED IN CLINIC

***Ismael Lares Asseff*[1,*], *Belén Juarez Tapia*[2] and *Christian J. Orea Sánchez*[2]**

[1]Centro Interdisciplinario de Investigación para el Desarrollo Integral Regional (CIIDIR), Instituto Politécnico Nacional, Durango, México
[2]Laboratorio de Farmacología, Instituto Nacional de Pediatría, Mexico City, México

ABSTRACT

The primordial objective of therapeutic optimization of any drug lies in reaching the plasmatic concentration within the therapeutic index (TI) that corresponds to the drug in such a way that the maximum pharmacological effect could be obtained. Such plasmatic concentration should produce its effect on getting to the therapeutic target in the site of biological action or biophase. In this site of biological action, the drug is simultaneously biotransformed in order to be excreted from the organism. Such excretion will depend on its pharmacokinetic and pharmacodynamic particularities. To get the precision and exactness of the plasmatic concentrations of a drug within the TI, it is necessary to know its pharmacokinetic characteristics as well as the effect which biological,

* Corresponding author: Ismael Lares Asseff. Instituto Politécnico Nacional, CIIDIR-Unidad Durango Calle Sigma 119. Fracc. 20 de noviembre II, Durango. Durango, Mexico, C.P. 34220. E-mail: ismaelares@yahoo.com.

physiological and physiopathological variables are going to exercise on the drug including the pharmacokinetic and/or pharmacodynamics interactions of other drugs or determined interactions of some food. To understand the pharmacokinetic process after the administration of a drug, it is important to consider the organism as a compartmental model which can be a monocompartmental or multicompartmental system. To have a knowledge of the destination of the drug in the organism, it is important to obtain its pharmcokinetic parameters in order to know what the organism does to the drug and then consider the application of pharmacokinetic in clinical practice. There is mathematical explanation which would permit the understanding and quantification of the kinetic processes experienced by a drug. Such mathematical basis uses the pharmacokinetic parameters as the volume of distribution (Vd), half-life elimination time (t1/2), depuration (Cl) and the area under the curve (ABC), among others. These parameters are normally determined by a first grade or lineal kinetic. Some of these kinetic processes could be saturated due to limited capacity during the absorption, distribution, metabolism and excretion that are defined by elimination kinetic of the order of zero or of Michaellis Menten. Each of the pharmacokinetic parameters has physiological explanation that will depend on the activity and/or functional capacity of the organs that participate in each of the pharmacokinetic processes. The pharmacokinetic parameters have biological explanation with therapeutic application where the objective is to design treatment regimen that would improve drug efficacy and safety in clinical practice.

INTRODUCTION

The most important thing of a therapeutic plan is to get the desired pharmacologic effect and this requires appropriate concentrations in the right target cell (where the binding to the receptors takes place) and their stay in the body for enough time to maximize therapeutic benefit with minimal side effects [1, 2]. When a drug is administered to a patient, the active substance undergoes a series of changes in the body that bring about the production of the pharmacological effect and to its eventual elimination. These changes involve certain vital body processes that lead to the dilution and distribution of the active substance to the different compartments, and finally its transformation to excretable metabolites [3]. Knowledge of the pharmacokinetic profile of any given drug and the variables that can change it, is quite useful in developing a rational dosing regimen to combat a disease and to prevent toxic effects [4]. Therefore, it is necessary to know the quantitative distribution based on the dose and route of administration. The time a drug persists in the body is determined by these two points – the dose and administration route.

The study of the kinetics of absorption, distribution and elimination of drugs in the body is an important part of pharmacokinetics. Concentration of the drug and its metabolites in the different compartments of the body, such as blood, tissues and excreta are measured in function of time and dose [3]. Although, the processes to determine the time course of both plasma concentrations and the activity of a drug in the body are extremely complex, these processes can be simplified by presenting the body as a system of limited compartments, from which a number of equations can be derived in order to obtain appropriate dosing regimens [4-6]. From their analysis, we can get parameters such as volume of distribution, clearance, half-life of elimination, which are indicators of the ability of biotransformation and distribution of drugs in the body. The application of these concepts in the therapeutic management of patients is known as clinical pharmacokinetics [6, 7].

MAIN ELEMENTS IN PHARMACOKINETICS

The mathematical explanation of the movement of a drug in the organism needs to be explained in response to a physiological reality as a simple and practical mathematical operation that demonstrates its applicability [5, 6]. To this purpose, the body is designed as a multi-compartment system in which, strictly speaking, each cell is a compartment which makes it almost impracticable for mathematical analysis and clinical application. Therefore, for the application of this mathematical analysis, the general rule only applies to few compartments [7]. In its physiological reality these compartments are separated by barriers according to their composition and conformation, which inhibit or facilitate the diffusion of the drug and where the physicochemical properties play an important role [6, 8, 9]. The amount of drug and/or its metabolites transported through membrane barriers will depend on the concentrations in the said compartments. It may happen that the quantity is not proportional to the drug concentration in the different compartments (i.e., saturation kinetics). If so, it means the existence of a limited capacity in the processes of transport, metabolism, or even elimination which could reflect on the treatment capacity or body clearance provoked by velocity, enzyme or membrane barrier [10].

Basics

As shown in Figure 1, it could be seen that immediately after delivering a substance intravenously as a single dose, there is a decrease in plasma concentrations due to its distribution, capture and biotransformation in: I) first the superficial tissues; II) the intermediate tissues which depletes the drug concentration even more; III) the various extravascular tissues throughout the body; IV) the deeper tissues and V) by a slower return of blood from the deep tissues that extends the duration of this decrease in the concentration. Upon completion this distribution, absorption or capture, tissue distribution equilibrium is established and this denotes the optimum time to estimate the volume of distribution in as much as the plasma concentration at zero time and the administered doses are known. The distribution volume depends on the drug and its property, and this varies from drug to drug [11, 12].

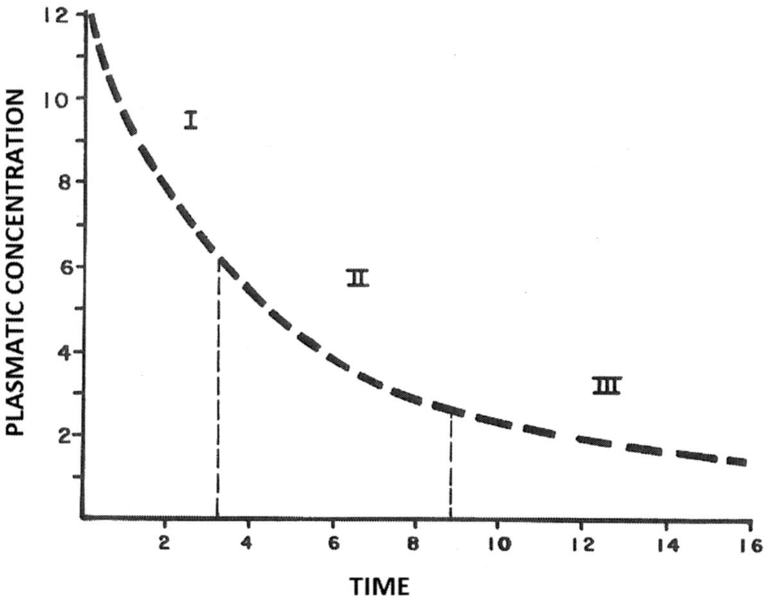

Figure 1. Decay curve of plasma concentrations of a drug administered intravenously. The segment (I) shows the distribution in superficial tissues. The segment (II) reflects the biotransformation and excretion, while the segment (III) represents the return of the drug from deep tissues.

MEANING OF THE VOLUME OF DISTRIBUTION IN THE CLINIC

The volume of distribution is a pharmacokinetic parameter to calculate the loading dose when it is necessary, and infer the location of the drug in the body [12]. Once a drug enters the bloodstream, it suffers a simultaneous distribution to body tissues and be removed by clearance organs (liver and kidneys). Only the free drug is distributed to extravascular tissues [13]. The acidic and neutral drugs bind to albumin, which has a higher binding capacity to drugs. Many basic (and some neutral) drugs bind to the protein of low capacity, -1-acid glycoprotein (AAG). This protein is very important because their serum concentrations are increased in conditions of stress, inflammatory and malignant diseases [14, 15].

The initial volume within which the drug is distributed (volume of distribution in the central compartment), includes blood volume (erythrocyte uptake, fixation to plasma proteins) and distribution in highly perfused parallel organs. It can exceed the physiological value when the drug is highly lipidsoluble or when it is rapidly fixed to skeletal tissue.

When the concentration of a substance reaches steady state, the volume of distribution at steady state (Vd_{SS}) or true volume is determined by the volume of blood (vascular volume) plus extravascular volume or tissue volume (total body water minus blood volume) times the ratio of drug binding to blood proteins and tissue [16] according to the following equation 1:

$$Vd_{SS} = Blood\ volume + \left(tissue\ volume\ \frac{free\ fraction\ of\ drug\ in\ blood}{free\ fraction\ of\ drug\ in\ tissue}\right) \quad (1)$$

As shown in this equation, drugs that have high affinity to plasma proteins will have a larger volume of distribution. Conversely, drugs with high affinity to blood proteins will have volumes of distribution approximately equal to blood volume.

Factors influencing the distribution of drugs include transport mechanisms (active or passive), the membrane permeability, the lipid solubility, the number of ionized molecules of the drug and the binding ability of the drug in serum [17].

Therefore, after a drug has entered into the systemic circulation, it undergoes multiple distribution processes which depend on their solubility in lipids, its pKa, the pH of body fluids, the binding ability to plasma proteins and tissue proteins, and differences in bloodstream. In organs that are highly perfused such as heart, liver, kidneys and endocrine glands; balance in the distribution is fast. While in adipose tissue and muscle which have a reduced blood supply, distribution equilibrium takes longer [12-17]. Phase 1, generally called distribution phase (Figure 1), corresponds to the peripheral tissue and it is usually the fastest step although, not instantaneous.

From the practical standpoint, the volume of distribution shows the relationship between the plasma drug levels (C) and the amount of drug in the body (D), because (equation 2):

$$C = D/Vd \qquad (2)$$

where: C = Concentration
D = Dose
Vd = Volume of distribution

Hence the doctor may change the dose (D) when the volume of distribution (Vd) generating a particular plasma level in an individual is known.

MEANING OF DRUG ELIMINATION IN THE CLINIC

Almost all drugs present a second phase (II) of slower decay of plasma levels (Figure 1). This phase is commonly called removal stage and involves both renal clearance and metabolic clearance. The half-life elimination ($t_{½\,el}$) is included within this phase and it is the time required for plasma concentration of a drug to be reduced to 50%, which can be determined for both compartments, the open model ($t_{½\,el}$) and two compartments ($t^1½\beta$). Therefore, the half-life of a drug is a useful clinical parameter to estimate the time a dose administered would remain in the body [18, 19].

The half-life of elimination is influenced by the volume of distribution (Vd) and clearance (t ½ = 0.693 Vd/Cl). The half-life of a drug may change as a result of alterations in plasma and tissue binding protein (for example, changes in the volume of distribution), or by changes in the function of the organs that eliminate drugs (for example, renal and/or liver failure) [18, 19].

The half-life of a drug has become a concept widely used in clinical pharmacology and medical therapeutics. Although, the half-life is an indicator of the removal processes, it has turned out to be very useful for determining appropriate dosing intervals at steady state (SS), either after administration by intravenous infusion, or orally in prolonged parameter.

Both in the case of one compartment model Kel and bicompartmental – β/2.303, the estimate of β can be obtained from the slope which corresponds to the exponential terminal phase and from there, it is possible to calculate the half-life (t ½) by applying the following equations (equation 3):

$$t_{1/2el} = \frac{0.693}{Kel} \quad o \quad t_{1/2} = \frac{0.693}{I?} \tag{3}$$

The first equation is used in the case of one-compartment open model and the second in two-compartment model.

MEANING OF TOTAL CLEARANCE IN THE CLINIC

In view of individual differences in enzyme capacity, it is reasonable to assume that the plasma half-life elimination will vary and will be different in each individual even when the same dose of a drug having metabolic clearance as their route of elimination is used [19-22]. When the available amount of metabolic enzymes is limited and plasma drug concentrations are high, removal capacity through this saturable metabolism approaches a constant value with the increase of plasma level [23]. The half-life of elimination of many drugs, due to their saturable metabolism becomes lengthened, hence, their chronic administration would generate toxic levels. In these cases, manifestations of toxicity doesn't keep a proportional relationship with dose because when the treatment is for a long time, even in small doses, it can provoke adverse effects [8, 21, 22].

Chemical transformation of a polar drug metabolism usually generates a polar molecule which is more soluble in bile and urine and it is easily excreted by these means. The liver is the most important organ for the metabolism of most drugs. These can be metabolized by phase I reactions (oxidation, reduction and hydrolysis) or by phase II reactions or synthetic: methylation, acetylation, sulfation and glucuronidation. Drugs are usually metabolized to inactive forms, but in some cases are metabolized into active forms [23, 24].

The removal efficiency of a drug by an organ is quantified by clearance. Liver efficiency (E) is determined by three physiological parameters: first by enzyme activity, second by the ability of the drug to bind to plasma proteins and third bloodstream speed through the liver as shown in equation 4 below:

$$Cl_H = Q\left(\frac{Cl_{int} \cdot f}{Q + Cl_{int} \cdot f}\right) \tag{4}$$

where Cl_H is hepatic clearance, f is the free fraction of the drug in blood, Cl_{int}, the intrinsic clearance of free drug, depending on the activity of drug metabolizing enzyme and the bloodstream to the liver [25, 26]. The complete derivation of the equation was performed by Shand et al. [27]. The intrinsic hepatic clearance is an expression of enzymatic activity in the liver. The magnitude of the intrinsic clearance depends on the strength and ability of interaction between the enzyme and drug, which varies from patient to patient and can change as a result of disease and drug interactions [26, 28]. In general terms, a drug with high intrinsic clearance would be more efficiently removed by the liver, and therefore have a high hepatic clearance. The ratio of extraction is given by the relation (Clint/Q + Clint) and varies from 0 to 1. When the drug has a high intrinsic clearance, the extraction ratio tends towards 1 and the clearance would be equivalent to hepatic bloodstream (Q) whereby the drugs are biotransformed rapidly depending essentially on Q. For this reason, they are said to be flow dependent.

On the other hand, there are drugs with low biotransformation; so their clearance is not dependent on bloodstream in the organ (Q) but on the intrinsic clearance and free drug. So, when intrinsic clearance is very low compared to blood flow, the extraction in the liver is low. For this, removing depends only on the enzymatic activity and the binding of the drug with proteins. In this case, drugs are said to be flow independent [28, 29].

Liver clearance or remove may change depending on the dose and concentration of the drug in cases where metabolic processes are of limited ability and the number of enzymes is limited. The theory of Michaelis Menten about enzyme kinetics shows that the metabolic speed of a drug is a function of two constants - Vmax and Km, and the concentration of free drug (equation 5) [29-31].

$$Rate\ metabolism = \frac{V_{max} \times free\ concentration}{Km + free\ concentration} \tag{5}$$

where V_{max} is the maximum rate of metabolism, which expresses the number of metabolic enzymes, while the constant of Michaelis (*Km*) represent the free concentration of serum drug in which metabolic rate is the half of the maximum value, $V_{max}/2$ [31].

MEANING OF DEEP COMPARTMENT IN CLINIC

Depending on the behavior in which plasma levels of a drug are reduced, it is possible to define two types of body compartments: the first is the shallow compartment in which plasma levels of a drug in peripheral tissues are practically proportional to the body, and the second is the deep compartment which refers to the bones, muscle tissue, connective tissue elements and the fetus or embryo [32].

Figure 2 illustrates the half-life of elimination where t ½ varies with time. While in the early hours of the drug, t ½ depends on the renal and metabolic elimination, and thereafter on the return from the deep tissues as shown in Figure 2. Also, it can be observed in the same Figure that the maximum concentration in the deep behavior is delayed without proportional relation with concentrations of the surface and central compartments.

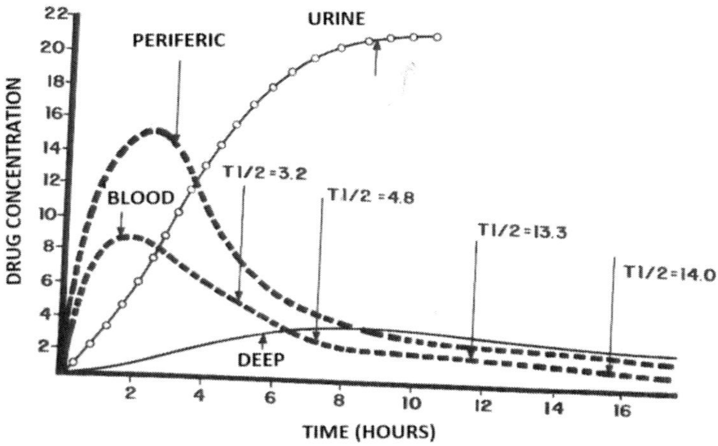

Garrett et al.

Figure 2. Shows the blood levels of drug in the surface and deep compartments and in urine, after first order absorption from the gastrointestinal tract. The surface compartment consists of tissue of rapid equilibrium, while the deep compartment are tissues of slow equilibrium.

Some drugs may have a slower decay (phase III). This phase is more evident in Figure 1 where the balance in the tissue distribution is not as fast. Sometimes, the extent of this deep compartment is quite important.

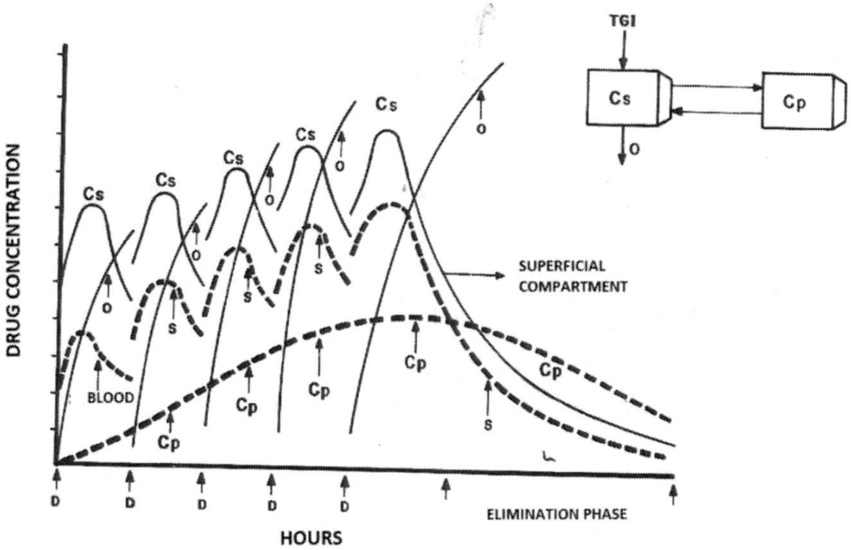

Garrett ER et al.

Figure 3. Shows the blood levels of drugs in superficial compartment (Cs), deep compartment (Cd) and urine after first-order absorption from the gastrointestinal tract (TGI).

So, in a regimen of prolonged treatment in patients with chronic illnesses, the body accumulates larger amount of the drug which is slowly removed in a prolonged way even when treatment is discontinued and this is due to slowness in the return of the drug from the deep compartment.

The best example of a deep compartment is represented by the embryo and fetus. As a result of the immaturity of their organs, there is an inability to metabolize drugs and/or its metabolites even in low concentrations, as well as transferring them to the organism of the mother and so, the only way to remove them is by degradation and excretion. This may explain why a drug may be harmful to the embryo or fetus and not to the mother [32].

Pharmacokinetics Applications in Clinic

The application of clinical pharmacokinetics goes beyond improving the effectiveness and safety of drugs. The magnitude in the kinetics of absorption, distribution and elimination of a drug varies from individual to individual however, the pharmacokinetic behavior of a drug is very similar in all humans.

Pharmacokinetic genetic variants can also be used to assess functional adequacy of different organs or as diagnosis to evaluate dynamic processes either of the type metabolic or pharmacokinetic [33].

Pharmacokinetic studies of certain drugs may be an indicative of the functional capacity of organs like the kidneys, liver, tissue binding capacity and/or permeability of membranes. The changes in pharmacokinetic parameters can be used as a warning to suspect a diagnosis at the time of disease manifestation or when there is clinical evidence of a functional disability. Individuals can be classified as fast or slow eliminators depending on their ability to remove a drug. So, based on this classification, physicians should apply a system of individualized treatment after an accurate and detailed kinetic analysis [34].

REFERENCES

[1] Buckley J, Birrell MA, Maher SA, Nials AT, Clarke DL, Belvisi MG. EP4 receptor as a new target for bronchodilator therapy. *Thorax* 2011; 66:1029-1035.

[2] Muller P and Milton MN. The determination and interpretation of the therapeutic index in drug development. *Nature Reviews Drug Discovery* 2012; 11: 751-761.

[3] Hutchinson LC, O'Brien CE. Changes in pharmacokinetics and pharmacodynamics in the elderly patient. *J Pharm Prac* 2007; 20:4-12.

[4] Mangoni AA, Jackson SH. Age-related changes in pharmacokinetics and pharmacodynamics: basic principles and practical applications. *Br J Clin Pharmacol* 2004; 57:6-14.

[5] Lüpfert C1, Reichl A. Development and application of physiologically based pharmacokinetic-modeling tools to support drug discovery. *Chem Biodivers* 2005; 2(11):14.

[6] Theil FP, Guentert TW, Haddad S, Poulin. Utility of physiologically based pharmacokinetic models to drug development and rational drug discovery candidate selection. *Toxicol Lett.* 2003;138(1-2):29-49.

[7] Withers RT, Laforgia J, Heymsfield SB. Critical appraisal of the estimation of body composition via two-, three-, and four-compartment models. *Am J Hum Biol* 1999;11:175-185.

[8] Krzyzanski W, Dmochowski J, Matsushima N, Jusko WJ. Assessment of dosing impact on intra-individual variability in estimation of parameters

for basic indirect response models. *J Pharmacokinet Pharmacodyn.* 2006;33(5):635-55.

[9] Benjamin B, Barman TK, Chaira T, Paliwal JK. Integration of physicochemical and pharmacokinetic parameters in lead optimization: a physiological pharmacokinetic model based approach. *Curr Drug Discov Technol.* 2010;7(3):143-53.

[10] Andersen ME. Saturable metabolism and its relationship to toxicity. *Crit Rev Toxicol.* 1981;9(2):105-50.

[11] Benet LZ, and Ronfeld RA. Volume terms in pharmacokinetics. *J Pharm Sci.* 1969;58:639.

[12] Riegelman S, Loo J, and Rowland M. Concept a volumen of distribution and posible errors in evaluation of this parameter. *J Pharm Sci.* 1968;57: 128-33.

[13] De Buck SS, Mackie CE. Physiologically based approaches towards the prediction of pharmacokinetics: in vitro-in vivo extrapolation. *Expert Opin Drug Metab Toxicol.* 2007;3(6):865-78.

[14] Israili ZH, Dayton PG. Human alpha-1-glycoprotein and its interactions with drugs. *Drug Metab Rev.* 2001; 33(2):161-235.

[15] Piafsky, KM: Disease-induced changes in the plasma binding of basic drugs. *Clin Pharmacokinet.* 1980;5(3):246-62.

[16] Benet LZ, Galeazzi RL. Noncompartmental determination of the steady-state volume of distribution. *J Pharm Sci.* 1979;68(8):1071-4.

[17] McNamara PJ, Leggas M. Drug Distribution. In: Hacker M, Messer II WS, Bachmann KA, editors. *Pharmacology: Principles and Practice.* First edition. San Diego, California US: Academic Press: 2009. P. 113-129.

[18] Paxton JW. Elementary pharmacokinetics in clinical practice I: drug absorption and disposition. *N Z Med J.* 1981; 94(694):304-6.

[19] Bauer LA. Primer on clinical pharmacokinetics. *Am J Hosp Pharm.* 1983; 40 (10):1637-41.

[20] Berlin NI, Berman M, Berk PD, Pang JM and Waldmann TA. The application of multicompartmental analysis to problems of clinical medicine. Combined clinical staff conference at the National Institutes of Health. *Ann Intern Med.* 1968;68(2):423-48.

[21] Temesvári M, Kóbori L, Paulik J, Sárváry E, Belic A, Monostory K. Estimation of drug-metabolizing capacity by cytochrome P450 genotyping and expression. *J Pharmacol Exp Ther.* 2012;341(1):294-305.

[22] Rowland M, Benet LZ, Graham GG. Clearance concepts in pharmacokinetics. *J Pharmacokinet Biopharm.* 1973;1(2):123-36.
[23] Dettli L. Capacity limited pharmacokinetics, a mechanism of drug toxicity (author's transl). *Arzneimittelforschung.* 1977; 27(96):1844-8.
[24] Brody BB, Gillette JR, and LaDu BN. Enzymatic metabolism of drugs and other foreign compounds. *Annu Rev Biochem*: 1958; 27(3):427-54.
[25] Conney AH. Drug metabolism and therapeutics. *N Engl J Med.* 1969; 280: 653-60.
[26] Wilkinson GR, Shand DG. Commentary: a physiological approach to hepatic drug clearance. *Clin Pharmacol Ther.* 1975; 18(4):377-390.
[27] Shand, DG: Recent advances in pharmacoklnetics. In: Shad D. G. P. Thurner eds. *Recent advances in Clinical Pharmacology*, Vol. 1 London Churchill Living Stone, 1978.1. 16.
[28] Callaghan R, Desmond PV, Mashford ML. Hepatic enzyme activity is the major factor determining elimination rate of high-clearance drugs in cirrhosis. *Hepatology.* 1993; 18(1):54-60.
[29] Rowland M, Tozer TN (1995). *Clinical Pharmacokinetics. Concepts and Applications.* Lippincott Williams and Wilkins. pp 161-167. ISBN 13: 978-0-6830-7404-8.
[30] Cornish-Bowden A. One hundred years of Michaelis–Menten kinetics. *Perspectives in Science.* 2015; 4: 3-9.
[31] Goudar CT, Sonnad JR, Duggleby RG. Parameter estimation using a direct solution of the integrated Michaelis–Menten equation. *Biochim Biophys Acta.* 1999; 1429: 377-383.
[32] Mirkin BL. Drug distribution in pregnancy. In: *Fetal Pharmacology*, edited by L.O. Boreus. Raven Press New York, 1973.
[33] Csajka C, Verotta D. Pharmacokinetic-pharmacodynamic modelling: history and perspectives. *J Pharmacokinet Pharmacodyn.* 2006; 33(3): 227-79.
[34] Wilkins JJ, Langdon G, McIlleron H, Pillai G, Smith PJ, Simonsson US. Variability in the population pharmacokinetics of isoniazid in South African tuberculosis patients. *Br J Clin Pharmacol* 2011;72(1):51-62.

In: Optimization of Drug Prescribing in Elderly ISBN: 978-1-63484-879-4
Editors: Juárez O. H. and Lares A. I.

Chapter 7

DIFFERENT METHODS USED TO DETERMINE THE PHARMACOKINETICS PARAMETERS

Juan Luis Chávez Pacheco[1,*], Hugo Juárez Olguín[2] and Ismael Lares Asseff[3]

[1]Laboratorio de Farmacología, Instituto Nacional de Pediatría, Mexico City, Mexico

[2]Laboratorio de Farmacología, Instituto Nacional de Pediatría, Mexico City, Mexico and Departamento de Farmacología, Facultad de Medicina, Universidad Nacional Autónoma de Mexico, México, D.F., Mexico

[3]Centro Interdisciplinario de Investigación para el Desarrollo Integral Regional (CIIDIR), Instituto Politécnico Nacional, Durango, México

ABSTRACT

The correct interpretation of what happens to a drug in the body after its administration, intra or extravascular route, resides on its movement with in the organism. This movement is known by information obtained from the pharmacokinetics profile of the drug expressed in terms of velocity. Hence, pharmacokinetics is defined as "the transformations a drug undergoes after its entrance into the organism." The pharmaco-

* Corresponding author: Juan Luis Chávez Pacheco. Laboratorio de Farmacología, Instituto Nacional de Pediatría. Avenida Imán # 1, 3er piso, Col Cuicuilco, CP 04530, Mexico D.F, Mexico. E-mail: jchavez_pacheco@hotmail.com.

kinetic parameters can only be obtained by means of mathematical models. However, there are various methods or models to calculate the pharmacokinetic parameters of a drug.

In the first place, it is important to consider the organism as a compartmental system with millions of compartments and then from a parsimonial point of view, find a simple mathematical model that would explain the pharmacokinetic processes from which we could derive mathematical equations that would define the pharmacokinetic parameters. Presently, there are two mathematical models the compartmental and non-compartmental. The compartmental model considers the velocity of entrance into, distribution in and egress of the drug from the organism, as well as the velocity of transference (or passage) from central compartment (more irrigated organs) to peripheral compartment (less irrigated organs) and vice versa. Fortunately in the present time, there are computer software which facilitate with high accuracy and speed the mathematical calculations to arrive at the pharmacokinetic parameters even if the data required to be adjusted to an open compartment model or to multi-compartment models an example of which may be the case of two-compartment open model.

This chapter is intended to take the reader step by step into what happens to a drug starting from the moment in which its plasma concentrations are obtained in function of time to graph the results in which the relations of drug concentrations versus time is expressed. The later would permit the definition of the compartmental model that best adjusts to the experimental data. Once the compartmental model is defined, the pharmacokinetic parameters are obtained and their clinical interpretations are carried out.

INTRODUCTION

When a drug is administered to an organism, it is distributed in a complex biological system that consists of cells. Although an individual biological unit, the cells are structured in tissues which are then organized into organ systems that make up the body.

On absorption of a drug, it is dispersed to a variety of spaces within the organs and body where it exerts its therapeutic effect by ligating to plasma and tissue proteins in the binding sites. And following its therapeutic actions, it is then removed from the body. The velocity of its distribution within the tissues depends on their tissue perfusion, the permeability of tissue, membranes to the particular drug and its relative separation between tissues and blood. Thus, in the absorption, distribution and elimination of a drug, the kinetics is the determinant factor and on these would depend the penetration of the drug molecules into the biological membranes to reach the site of pharmacological action [1-3].

In order to simplify this complexity and make quantitative analysis, it is necessary to understand the mechanisms of movement of drugs in the body and its expression as mathematical phenomena to estimate the rate and speed. The principal processes observed in pharmacokinetics are typified as first-order, zero-order and limited capacity (Figure 1). The human body can be considered as a homogeneous system by way of a compartment (Figure 2) or as a multi-compartment system (Figure 3) in which the administered drugs are distributed at different rates in different body fluids and tissues [4]. These compartments have an anatomical boundary and each consists of a particular tissue type, so that the number of compartments, which can be defined in a particular case, depends on the number of areas with different permeation rates for a drug [5] (Figure 3). From the experimental point of view, it is difficult and very complex to show more than three compartments, and sometimes, even three compartments are difficult.

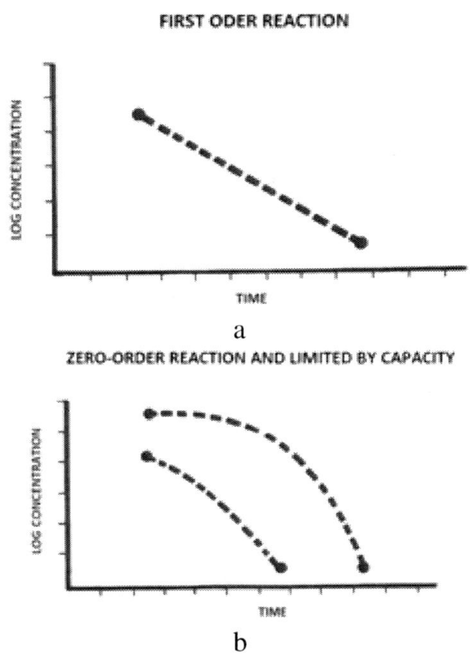

Figure 1. Illustrates the ratio expressed as first order reactions (a), zero order (b), and Michaellis Menten kinetics (b).

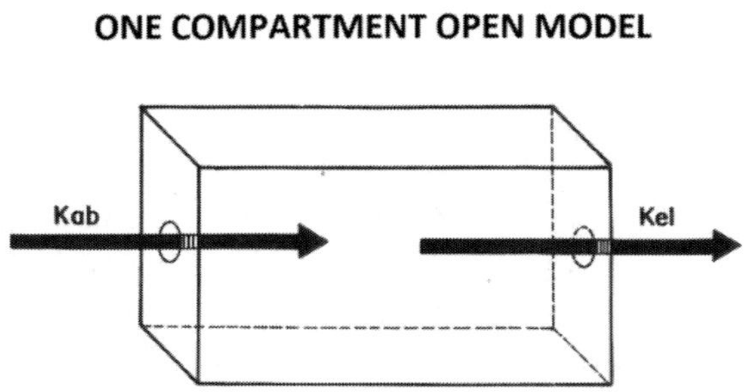

Figure 2. Schematic representation of one-compartment model with constant input speed, Ka, absorption rate and elimination rate constant, Kel.

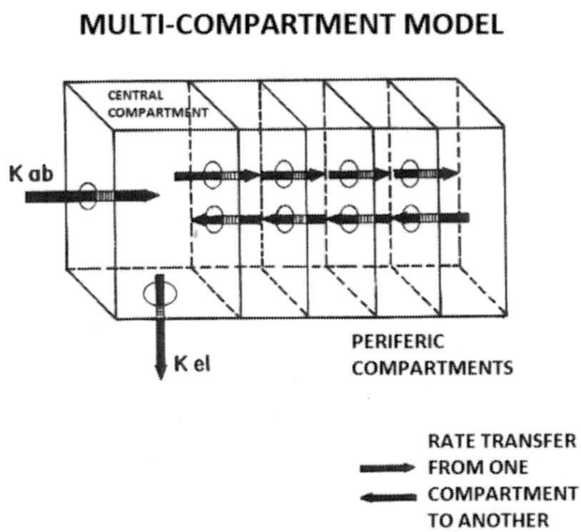

Figure 3. Schematic representation of a multi-compartment open model with input speeds, Kab. Transfer rates between compartments, and elimination rate, Kel.

From the pharmacokinetic point of view, it is important that the plasma concentration of a drug must conform to mathematical equations, which represent the passage of drugs and their metabolites through compartmental models of the experimental data observed. Although every drug and every individual who is given a drug possesses properties and characteristics which determine a pharmacokinetic compartment and this may vary from individual to individual or from one drug to another. Certain general principles of pharmacokinetic data manipulation must be applied in such a way that this will result in a precise description of the available drug which has major applications in the clinic, especially with drugs considered at high risk in their therapeutic management [6].

Some assumptions must be taken into account when using the compartmental models and mathematical equations to define the dynamic behavior of a drug in the body.

The first of these assumptions is that drugs entering the organism should only do so through the central compartment, and their removal is only from this compartment.

The second is that there is a reversible transfer between the central and the peripheral compartment.

The third, lies on the output where it is assumed that the output of drugs from all compartments in the system is described by first order kinetics. This means that the rate at which a drug is removed from a compartment is directly proportional to the drug concentration in the same compartment [6, 11]. However, drugs having kinetics of zero order, where the enzyme systems that metabolize the drug for biotransformation and elimination from the body are saturated are exception in this regard.

Figure 4 describes each of the steps required for the analysis of the time course of plasma concentrations of a drug administered to an individual, and the pharmacokinetic parameters that can be used for its evaluation and design of less toxic therapeutic regimens that are more effective.

With the advent of recent analytical techniques such as high performance liquid chromatography (HPLC), gas chromatography, radioimmunoassay and enzyme immunoassay, it is possible to have a more accurate measurement and higher sensitivity that will detect extremely small quantities of drugs and their metabolites in biological fluids. These techniques have made it possible to study and characterize the time course of absorption, distribution, metabolism and excretion of many drugs.

The obtained concentrations are plotted on graph paper and the maximum plasma concentration (Cpmax), the time in which the aforementioned maximum concentration Tmax is reached, and the area under the curve (AUC), obtained by the concentration versus time is calculated (Figure 5).

The plasma levels which should be plotted on millimetric paper considering the Cartesian system, where the y-axis corresponds to the observed concentrations, which are expressed in the units in which the measurements are made and x-axis is plotted over time, which can be expressed in minutes, hours or days depending on the sampling time of a particular drug.

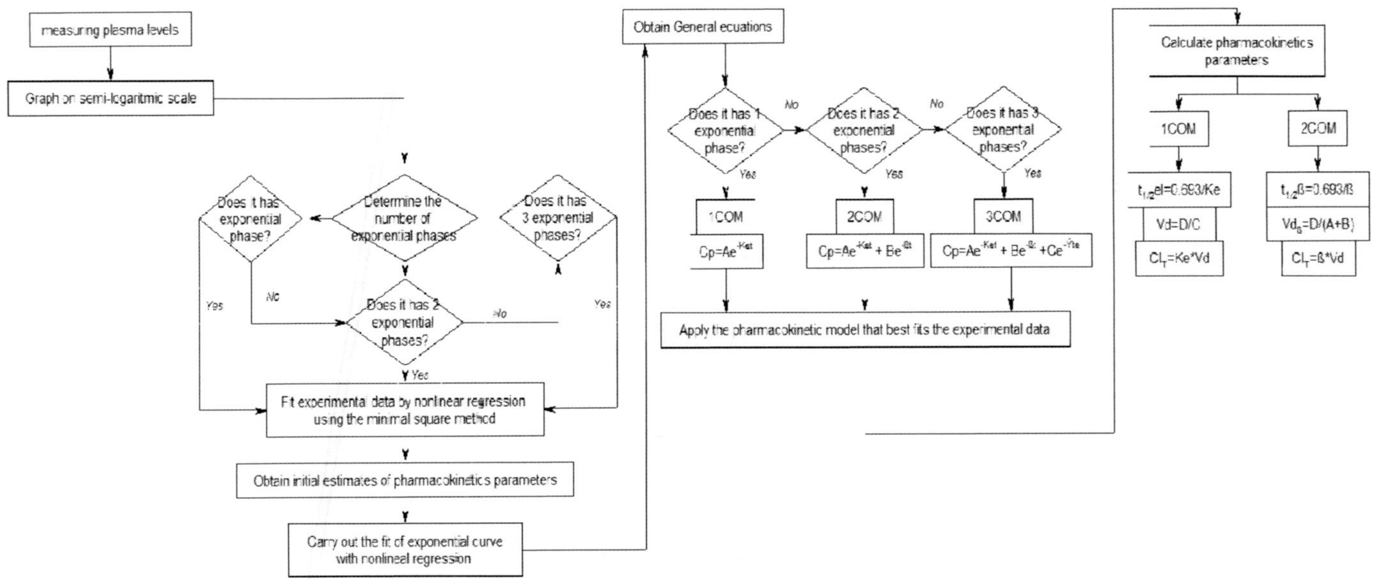

Figure 4. Flow diagram that describes the steps necessary to carry out pharmacokinetic calculations.

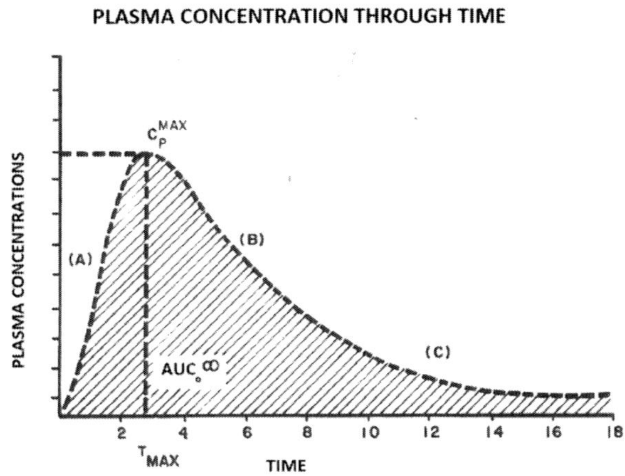

Figure 5. Schematic diagram of AUC of the levels of a drug levels in blood versus time. AUC → ∞ and Cpmax is the maximum peak and Tmax is the maximum time in which Tmax is reached after an oral administration of a single dose. (A) Absorption phase, (B) distribution phase, (C) Stage of elimination, until the time when the last sample was taken.

Figure 5 shows the plasma concentration profile versus time after administration: A is the absorption stage, Cpmax is the maximum plasma concentration, Tmax is the time at which the maximum plasma concentration is obtained, B is the distribution phase and C is the elimination phase in which biodegradation mechanisms of liver and/or kidney are involved. It is also possible to calculate the area under the curve from the zero time to infinity (AUC → ∞), which indicates the time of the drug in the body. The area under the curve of blood levels versus time is a measure of the total amount of drug in the body.

The AUC can be calculated in two ways; the first approach is to cut the sheef of paper in the area bounded by this curve and then weighs it. The weight obtained is then transformed into quantity measurements. The other way is to use the trapezoidal rule in calculating the area beginning from zero time (time = 0) to the time the last blood sample is taken (t = x) [7]. Thus, AUC → ∞ is determined in two steps:

a) First, calculate the area from time = 0

Then calculate the area under the curve of the last concentration obtained until infinitum. The area under the curve from 0 to ∞ (from zero to infinity) =

the sum of the areas of all the trapezoids between points 2 blood samples and their respective times [8] (Figure 6).

i.e.,

$$AUC \rightarrow \infty = AUC_{0\rightarrow}tx + AUCtx\rightarrow\infty \quad (1)$$

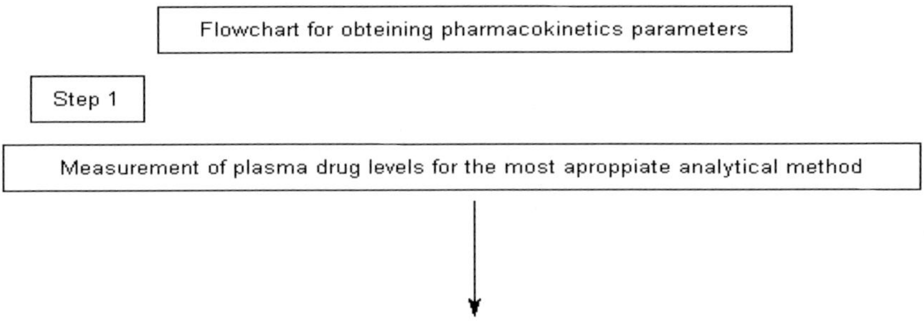

Figure 6. Step 1. Flow Chart to Obtain Pharmacokinetic Parameters.

b) The second step is to obtain the area of the curve under the last blood sample taken C over the time (X) to the infinitum AUC (x→∞) (Figure 7).

This is calculated as follows:

$$AUC(x \rightarrow \infty) = C\ (x)/Kel \text{ or } \beta\ (ug/ml).h \quad (2)$$

Therefore, the total area under the curve from zero to infinity (AUC o→∞) is the sum of equations 1 and 2:

$$AUC\ (o\rightarrow\infty) = \Sigma[(Cn + Cn + 1)/2)\ (tn + 1 - tn)] + C\ (x)/Kel \text{ or } \beta \quad (3)$$

From the total area under the curve from zero to infinity, we can calculate the clearance (CL_T) and the apparent volume of distribution (Vd) as respectively shown in equations 4 and 5 below.

$$CL_{tot} = D/AUC_{0\rightarrow\infty} \quad (4)$$

$$Vd = D/AUCo\rightarrow\infty.\beta \text{ or } k_{el} \quad (5)$$

where D is the dose and AUC is the area under the curve of concentration vs. time graph.

When the drug is administered extravascularly, the amount of administered dose (D) must be multiplied by the absolute bioavailability (F).

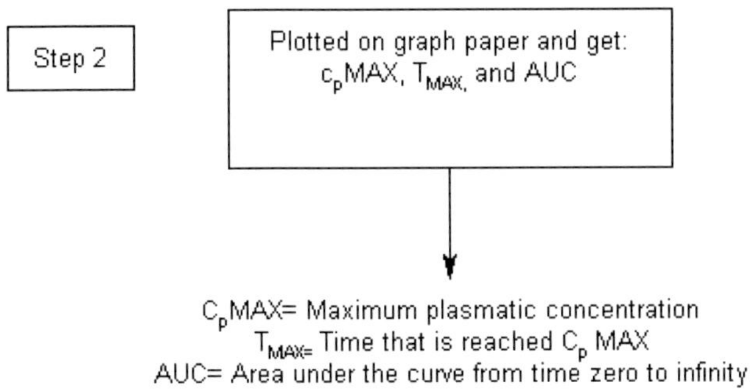

Figure 7. Step 2.

When the administration is carried out intravenously, the above values can be obtained with the exception of absorption phase, the maximum plasma concentration (Cpmax), and the time at which the said concentration is reached (Tmax).

Like on graph paper, experimental plasma concentrations are plotted and expressed in units of mass/volume (mg/ml, mg/100 ml, ug/ml, units/ml, etc.) (y-axis) versus time (x-axis). The purpose of the profile graphs (concentration versus time using semilog paper) is to visually determine the number of exponential phases during the decline of the concentrations (Figure 8). The number of phases indicates the compartmental model that best explains the behavior following the experimental values. Therefore, the first step in making decision on whether to choose any pharmacokinetic model (one or multi-compartment) is to inspect the graph of concentration against time.

To make this decision, a straight line connecting approximately all points of the terminal phase of the slope, according to the proposed terminal by Ritschell WA. Method [9], is drawn until the Y-axis or its intersection with the ordinate. The pharmacokinetic model to be chosen depends on the side of the line (above or below) in which the more concentration points are found. In this regard, if more of the concentration points the below the line, it applies that the graph is open compartment model. On the contrary, i.e., if concentrations points are markedly above this line, it must be assumed that the graph represents a multi-compartmental model of two or more compartments as schematically shown in the graphs in Figure 9. This inspection method (traced by eye) allows us to have an approach to the choice of the mathematical model to explain better the pharmacokinetic behavior. At this moment we are in a position to propose a mathematical model through which the pharmacokinetic parameters are obtained.

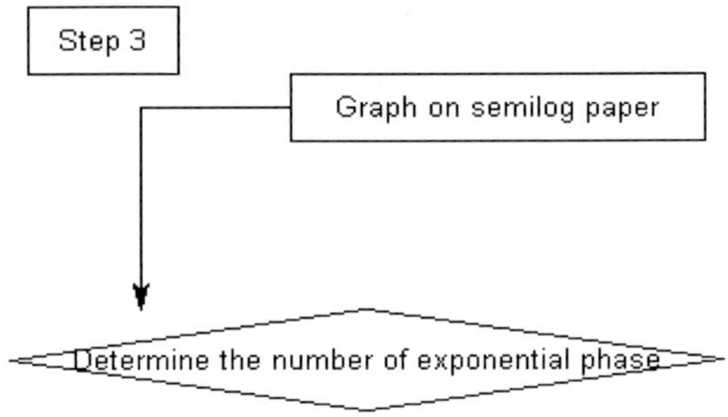

Figure 8. Step 3.

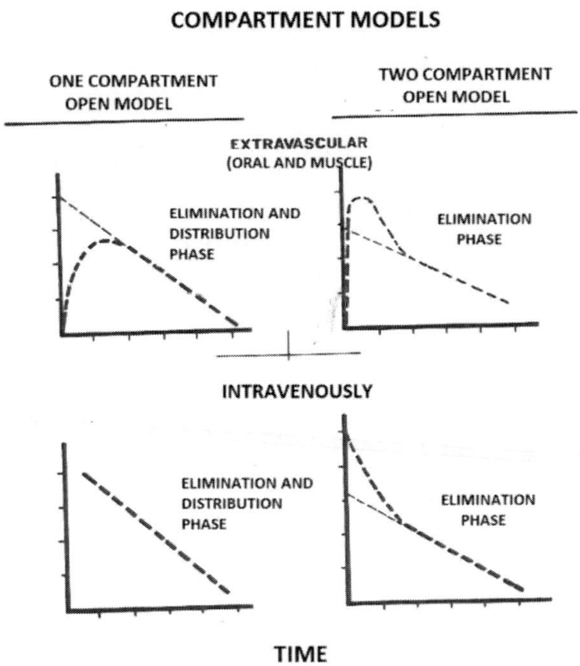

Figure 9. Schematic diagram for choosing the pharmacokinetic model. Source: Ritschel, WA: *Graph Approach to Clinical Pharmacokinetics* 2nd. Ed. J.R.J. Prous Publishers. Barcelona, 1984, p. 20.

The next step is to make the mathematical test to check if the proposed pharmacokinetic model is the one that best explains the observed concentration profiles, considering the successive steps, once it has tentatively defined the number of exponential phases.

Step 4: Setting the experimental data to a nonlinear model by the method of least squares (Figure 10).

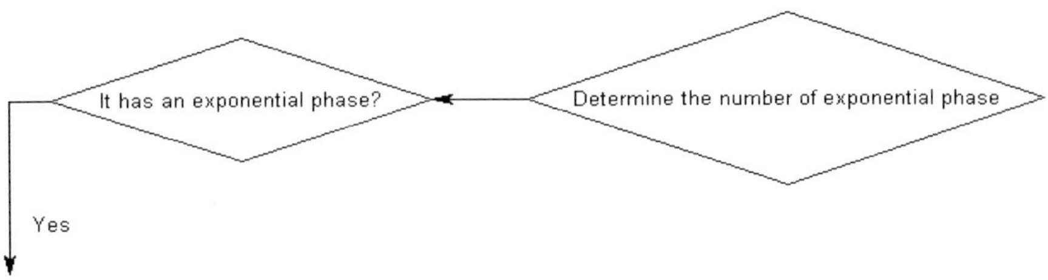

Figure 10. Step 4.

There is a more objective and accurate method consisting in transforming all concentration values in their logarithms and then calculate regression lines of each exponential phase by the method of least squares described in the books of statistics [8, 9]. The detailed description of the mathematical calculations of each model are described below.

On the basis of the number predetermined by the method of inspection of the exponential phase, we are in a position to suspect the pharmacokinetic model that best explains the experimental data through the general equations describing the theoretical behavior of the plasma concentration versus time which define the pharmacokinetic model.

As noted, it is desirable to determine whether the profile of plasma concentration versus time forms one, two, or more exponential phases that define the compartmental model and carry out the calculations of the method of least squares that allow to choose the pharmacokinetic model. Such studies can be done both manually and/or with the help of a personal computer. Currently there are programs in minicomputers, microcomputers and computers with large capacity (WINONLINE) [10] to successfully carry out this operation. Therefore, we can apply any of these technologies if available or depending on the level of attention required.

In minicomputers, programs leading to initial estimates of pharmacokinetic parameters [9] are used. After obtaining initial estimates, a more complex program, such as the nonlinear regression, uses the Gauss-Newton algorithm [10].

Following Figure 4 step 3, we can determine whether it has an exponential phase after getting a linear relationship of the data obtained in the study, as it shows in Figure 11.

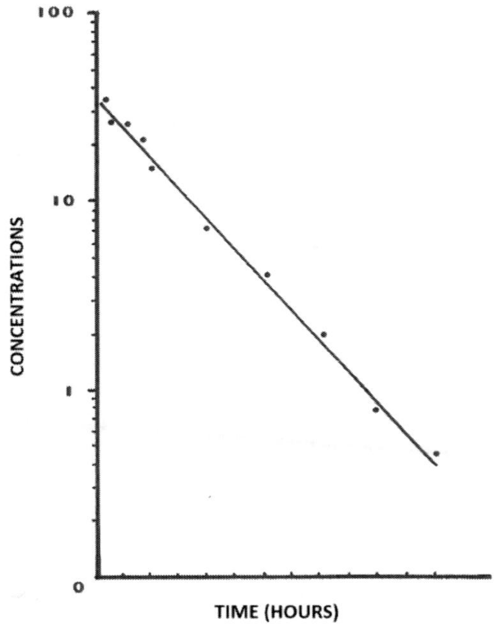

Figure 11. Plasma concentration declining curve in function of time in a semi-logarithmic scale defined by the following mono-exponential equation.

Step 5. Check the number of exponentials (Figure 12)

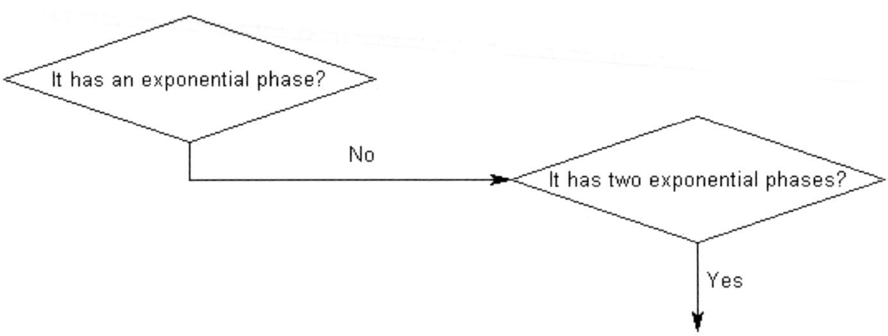

Figure 12. Step 5.

If the experimental data fit to one compartmental model [11, 12], initial estimates of the exponential curve obtained for the general equation of a compartment open model are done.

$$Cp = Ae^{-Kel.t} \quad (6)$$

where: A: is the intercept of the extrapolated slope, Kel: is the elimination rate constant, $t_{1/2el}$: is time of half life, Cp: corresponds to the natural logarithm of plasma concentration.

If the experimental data do not conform to a one-compartment model, then we proceed to determine whether the curve is composed of two exponential phases describing a two-compartment model and graph the data in the form as shown in Figure 13.

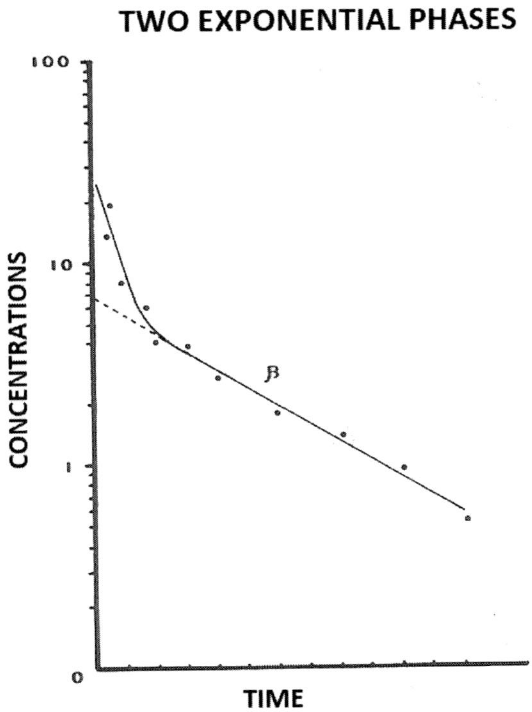

Figure 13. Classic open two-compartment model after a single intravascular administration.

The β phase represents not only the net effect of removing the medicament but drug movement in and out of different tissues. The same considerations can be applied to the rapid decline phase called α and corresponds to the distribution stage. This line is obtained by subtracting the values of the observed concentrations from the corresponding concentrations of the extrapolated line of the α phase at time zero. The residuals are plotted on the same graph and a line is obtained after performing the best fit. The slope of this line defines α as the rate of constant distribution.

Extrapolating this line to zero is the intercept time A, and phase B determines extrapolated intercept B. Thus the plasma concentration at zero time (Co) is the sum of the intercepts of A + B.

The theoretical plasma concentration at any time is the sum of the exponential processes so that the general equation defining the model is as follows (equation 7):

$$Cp = Ae^{-\alpha . t} + Be^{-\beta . t} \quad (7)$$

Mathematical manipulations to this equation make possible to obtain some constants [8, 9]. Note that all constants (A, B, α and β) are hybrid coefficients depending on the combination of k12, k21, V1 and V2 and the administered dose [6].

General algebraic manipulation of the equation would lead to the derivation of the following relationships:

$$Vd = Dose/A + B \quad (8)$$

$$\alpha + \beta = k_{12} + k_{21} + K_{10} \quad (9)$$

$$\alpha \text{ x } \beta = k_{12} \text{ x } K_{10} \quad (10)$$

And from B the following expression is obtained:

$$k_{21} = (A \text{ x } \beta) + (B \text{ x } \alpha)/A + B \quad (11)$$

$$K_{12} = \alpha + \beta - k_{21} - k_{10} \quad (12)$$

$$k_{10} = \alpha \text{ x } \beta/k_{21} \quad (13)$$

Micro-constant determines by equations 11, 12, and 13 would allow an assessment of the relative contribution of the processes of distribution and elimination profile of a drug concentration with respect to time. It can also help clarify the mechanism of drug interactions and the effects of disease, age, genetic influence, clinical condition, and disposition of the drug [11-14].

Finally, plasma clearance or clearance is obtained through the elimination rate constant and the volume of distribution Vd by applying the equation below:

$$CL_T = Kel \times Vd \tag{14}$$

The two-compartment model can be expanded to contain additional compartments, which can be described mathematically as the sum of many exponential functions as the number of compartments increases [4-6].

If the experimental data do not conform to a two-compartment model, then we proceed to determine whether the curve is composed of three or more exponential phases describing a multi-compartment model as exemplified in Figure 15, once the experimental data are plotted.

In this case the initial parameter estimates of the tri-exponential curve was also calculated using the method of waste, in order to obtain a general equation describing the 3-compartment open model.

$$Cp = Ae^{-\alpha \times t} + Be^{-\beta \times t} + Ce^{-\gamma \times t} \tag{15}$$

The calculation of a larger three-compartment model is very complex. For this reason, it is better to opt for the principle of parsimony and choose the simplest model that explains the phenomenon [6].

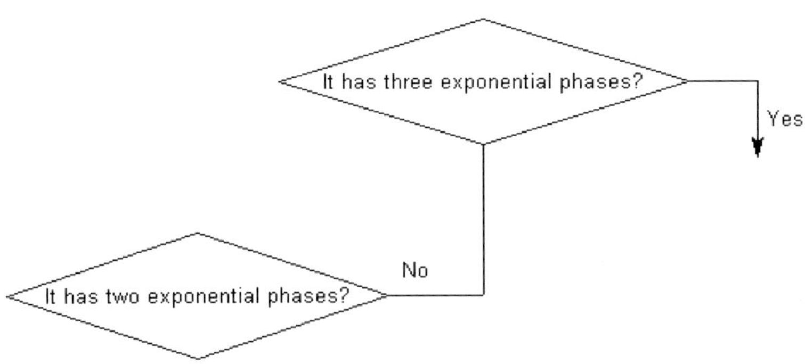

Figure 14. Step 6.

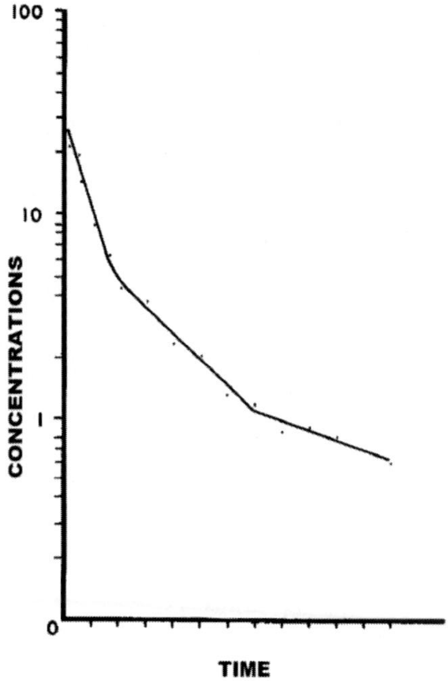

Figure15. Concentrations of a drug versus time in a semi-logarithmic scale; decay curve fits a tri-exponential function corresponding to a three-compartment open model.

In Figure 15 is shown an example, In this case a rapid initial phase (distribution), and the two end stages through which the lines of the elimination of peripheral compartments (one surface and another deep) pass are observed.

Step 7: To obtain the general equations describing the pharmacokinetic model (Figure 16).

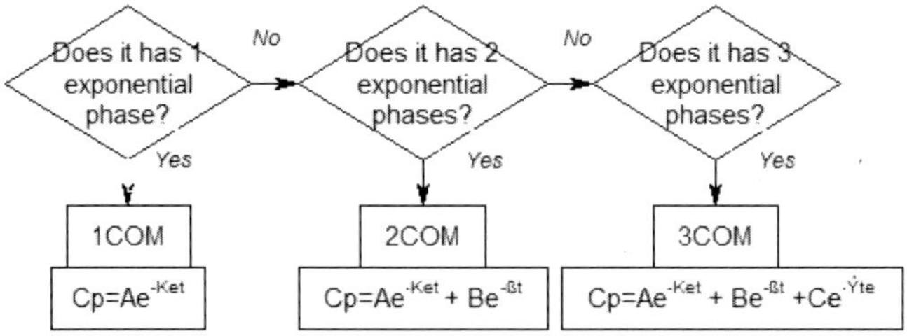

Figure 16. Step 7.

Step 8: Apply the selection criteria for pharmacokinetic model.

Once the general equation describing the pharmacokinetic behavior is derived, apply the criteria to choose the exponential curve that best explains the experimental data. In this case, statistical methods as x^2 test, to determine the goodness of fit [15]; or an analysis of covariance can be used.

For pharmacokinetic data, Akaike criterion [16] has been proposed. This method has similarity with the x^2 test and only considers the number of compartmental pharmacokinetic parameters depending on the model.

Step 9: Calculation of the pharmacokinetic parameters (Figure 17).

Having chosen a mathematical model that best explains the experimental data; we proceed to calculate some of the pharmacokinetic parameters useful for the design of a treatment regimen, as noted below (Figure 17):

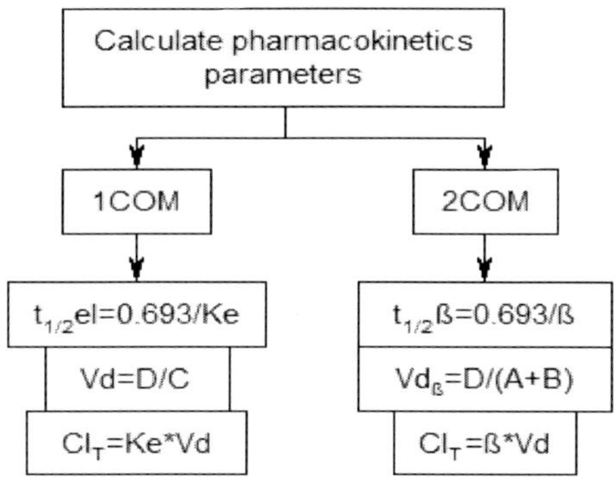

Figure 17. Step 9.

APPLYING THE CONCEPTS TO EVALUATE PHARMACOKINETIC AND OPTIMIZATION OF THERAPEUTIC REGIMENS

Since variability in the intra- and interindividual pharmacokinetic behavior are not the exception but the rule and depends on many factors including age, nutritional status, smoking, alcoholism, time of administration, disease states and genetic aspects, etc. individualized treatment regimen will be required. Such treatment scheme can be obtained through pharmacokinetic knowledge of a particular individual such as a patient at high risk of toxicity or a patient that uses drugs with high risk of producing side effects due to their narrow therapeutic index. Thus, application of pharmacokinetic principles would help to achieve the desired plasma concentration.

The relationship between plasma concentration and the clinical response has been demonstrated for different drugs [17, 18]. Other studies relating to this are aimed at defining the concentrations associated with a higher incidence of toxic effects.

DRUG ACCUMULATION

Most drugs are administered in repeated doses for a prolonged time or chronically. If doses are administered at a very long intervals (greater than the elimination half-life of the drug), or if the clearance is very rapid, the drug disappears from the body before the next dose is administered. In contrast, when the administration is at smaller interval (smaller than the half-life of elimination of the drug), drug accumulation will occur until a constant plateau, that is, an equilibrium state is reached. An equilibrium state is depicted at that point when the delivery rate and the removal rate are the same. As shown in Figure 18, it is clear that for a multiple dose regimen, a certain amount of the drug remains in the body when the next dose is administered. The time required to obtain a steady state depends on the half-life of elimination. To get drug concentrations in equilibrium state requires at least four half-lives [19, 20].

The accumulation of a drug, as already mentioned, depends on the relative frequency of dosing intervals, time and elimination half-life (t½ el): if the proportion of range management to the half-life elimination $t_{1/2el}$ is smaller, the accumulation is more important. Conversely, if the ratio is larger, the accumulation is less; or there may be significant fluctuations between the maximum plasma concentrations ($Cmax_{ss}$) and the minimum steady state concentrations ($Cmin_{ss}$). The amplitude of fluctuations is a function of $t_{½el}$ and the larger the proportion of $t_{½el}$, the greater the fluctuation.

The most useful equation in pharmacokinetics for predicting the concentrations achieved with a treatment regimen established gives birth to pharmacokinetic data, the average concentration at a steady state (Css) which does not itself represent an average value between the values of maximum and minimum concentrations. This useful equation is as shown below:

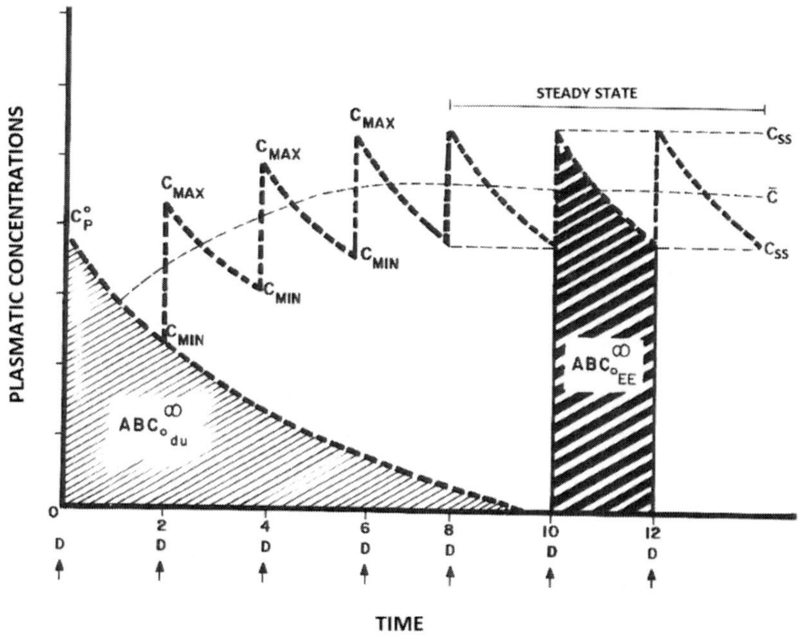

Figure 18. Blood levels of a drug against time, to demonstrate the accumulation at steady state (One-compartment open model) where: ABCo → ∞ = the area under the curve from zero to infinity, obtained after a single dose of medication. ABCo ∞ ee corresponds also to the area under the curve from zero to infinity in the steady state. $Cmax_{ss}$ = is the maximum plasma concentration at steady state. $Cmin_{ss}$ = is the minimum plasma concentration at steady state. Source: Ritschel WA: *Handbook of Basic Pharmacokinetics* 2nd. Of Drug Intelligence Publications. Inc. Hamilton, Illinois, 1980, p. 259.

$$Css = F \times D/Kel \times Vd = F \times D/Cl_T \quad (16)$$

As can be seen, Css is different depending on the pharmacokinetic parameters such as total clearance (CL_T) and drug input rate Q [19, 20].

Dose Adjustment for a Therapeutic Regimen of Repeated Administration

In this case, the drug accumulation is the result of either orally or parenterally repeated administration of the drug at regular intervals in chronic form. The accumulation of the drug is governed by the same factors controlling accumulation by continuous intravenous infusion, such as input speed and drug clearance. As noted above, each intermittent administration determines the peaks (highest concentrations) and the valleys (lowest levels) reached (Figure 18) applying the aforementioned criteria to determine the plasma concentration at steady state through the equation 16.

If we desire to reach the therapeutic concentrations rapidly, the loading dose to be administered intravenously should be calculated using equation 17:

$$LD = Vd \times Mc \quad (17)$$

where: LD = Loading dose, Vd = Volume of distribution, Mc = Mean Concentration.

To maintain the desired plasma concentrations within the therapeutic range, the amount of medication lost has to be replaced in such a way that if the total body clearance (CL_T) and/or renal clearance (CL_R) is known, the maintenance dose can be calculated as follows (equation 18):

$$DM = CL_T \times Css \quad (18)$$

where Css is the desired plasma concentration and CL_T is the total body clearance.

If administrations are made orally, the bioavailability of the drug must be considered and the following correction is made (equation 19):

$$DM = CL_T \times Css/F \quad (19)$$

Sustained Therapeutic Concentrations

Given the multiplicity of factors that influence the plasma concentrations achieved with a treatment regimen, which can lead to treatment failure, either by reaching levels that are below actual levels or reaching toxic levels; it is necessary to apply the pharmacokinetic knowledge in order to obtain a more accurate approximation of the desired plasma concentrations.

A strategy for therapeutic success can be achieved through the empirical approach, which does not require individualized treatment regimen but the recommended basic drug tables and treaties of pharmacology doses. The results are great variations in plasma concentrations and clinical response. However, when drugs with a narrow therapeutic index are handled, there is the risk of toxicity and/or treatment failure.

When it is not possible to lay hand on the pharmacokinetic parameters of a particular patient, the pharmacokinetic parameters in the literature, which corresponds to individuals with the same biological similarities and/or pathological features that best match the individual in question is obtained. Such exercise is good and could render better result than ignoring them. These elements will contribute in establishing an evaluation system for feedback [21, 22] between the desired concentrations and the administered dose. So, the monitoring of the plasma levels would determine the success or failure of a treatment regimen and this can be evaluated as shown in Figure 19.

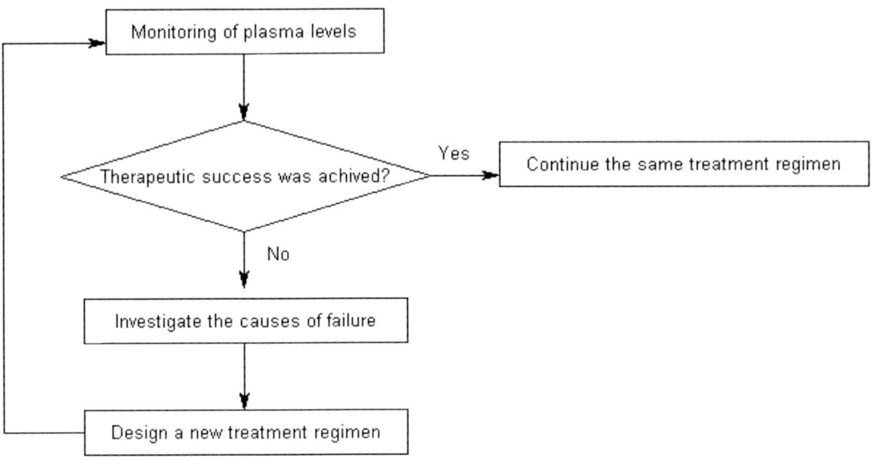

Figure 19. Procedure to therapeutic drug monitoring.

It is a process that permits the achievement of the therapeutic success by successive approximations with the feedback model or "Feedback." In short, the system requires the following:

a) Administering a dose designed to achieve the therapeutic levels and to maintain it below toxic levels or half the therapeutic range for the particular drug.
b) Plasma concentrations after an appropriate period should be monitored with the prescribed regimen. The time to take the sample to perform therapeutic monitoring should be when the concentration is at

steady state. This is different for each drug and should be done after 5 half-lives, which varies according to the drug in question.

c) If the dose is inadequate, the causes that lead to failure are investigated, and a new treatment regimen is designed.
d) Once the dose is adjusted, the plasma concentration is again determined and the clinical response is re-evaluated until the desired therapeutic effect is achieved.

REFERENCES

[1] Capaldi RA. Dynamic model of cell membranes. *Sci Am* 1974; 230(3): 26-33.

[2] Wagner JG. Biopharmaceutics: gastrointestinal absorption aspects. *Antibiot Chemother*. 1964; 12: 53-84.

[3] Paton WDM. A Theory of Drug Action Based on the Rate of Drug-Receptor Combination. *Proc R Soc Lon B*. 1961; 154:21-69.

[4] Levy G, Gibaldi M, and Jusko WJ. Multi-compartment pharmacokinetic models and pharmacologic effects. *J Pharm Sci* 1969; 58(4): 422-424.

[5] Riggs DS. A critical primer - The mathematical approach to physiological problems, M.I.T. Press, Cambridge, Mass. 1967, p. 193.

[6] Berlin NI, Berman M, Berk PD, Phang JM, Waldmann TA. The application of multicompartmental analysis to problems of clinical medicine. Combined clinical staff conference at the National Institutes of Health. *Ann Intern Med*. 1968; 68(2): 423-48.

[7] Myerson J, Green L, and Warusawitharana M. Area under the curve as a measure of discounting. *J Exp Anal Behav*. 2001; 76(2): 235-243.

[8] Hanley JA, and McNeil BJ. The meaning and use of the area under a receiver operating characteristic (ROC) curve. *Radiology*. 1982;143(1): 29-36.

[9] Ritschell WA. *Handbook of the Basic Pharmacokinetics*. 2nd Updated Ed. Chapter 17, Drug Intelligence Publications, Hamilton, Ill. 1982, pp. 208-218.

[10] Win-Nonlin program, Standard edition, version 2.1. Mountain View, CA: Scientific Consultation Inc.; 1991.

[11] Berman M, and Schoenfeld R. Invariants in experimental data on linear kinetics and the formulation of models. *J Appl Physics* 1956;27: 1361-70.

[12] Gerlowski LE, and Jain RK. Physiologically based pharmacokinetic modeling: principles and applications. *J Pharm Sci.* 1983;72(10):1103-1125.
[13] Benet LZ. Editor: The effect of disease states on drug pharmacokinetics. 123rd Annual Meeting, American Pharmaceutical Association, New Orleans, Louisiana, 1976.
[14] Evans W E, Schentag J J, Jusko W J, Harrison H, eds. (1992). In: Evans W E, Schentag J J, eds. *Applied Pharmacokinetics: Principles of Therapeutic Drug Monitoring*, 3rd edn. Vancouver: Applied Therapeutics.
[15] Castilla L, Cravioto J. (1991). Estadística Simplificada para la Investigación en Ciencias de la Salud (Simplified Statistics for Research in Health Sciences). Editorial Trillas, México, pp. 174-181.
[16] Yamoaka K, Nakagawa T, Uno T. Application of Akaike's information (AIC) in the evaluation of linear pharmacokinetics equations. *J Pharmacokinet Biopharm.* 1978; 6:165 175.
[17] Golan, D. "Principles of Pharmacology: The Pathophysiologic Basis of Drug Therapy." 2nd ed. LWW, 2008.
[18] Muller PY and Milton MN. The determination and interpretation of the therapeutic index in drug development. *Nature Reviews Drug Discovery.* 2012; 11:751-761.
[19] Smith IL, Schentag JJ. Noncompartmental determination of the steady-state volume of distribution during multiple dosing. *J Pharm Sci.* 1984; 73(2): 281-2. *Pharm Res.* 1998 Nov;15(11):1796-8.
[20] Hauck WW, Tozer TN, Anderson S, Bois FY. Considerations in the attainment of steady state: aggregate vs. individual assessment. *Pharm Res.* 1998; 15(11): 1796-8.
[21] Birkett DJ. Pharmacokinetics made easy 9: Non-linear pharmacokinetics. *Aust Prescr* 1994;17:36-8.
[22] Lewis BS, Halkin H, Peck C, Rosenberg B, and Melmon ID. Improved Computer-Assisted Digoxin Therapy: A Method Using Feedback of Measured Serum Digoxin Concentrations. *Ann Intern Med.* 1975; 82(5): 619-627.

In: Optimization of Drug Prescribing in Elderly ISBN: 978-1-63484-879-4
Editors: Juárez O. H. and Lares A. I.

Chapter 8

PHARMACOKINETICS STUDIES AND THE INTERPRETATION OF DRUG LEVELS IN STEADY STATE

Gabriela Pérez Guillé[1,*], Belén Juárez Tapia[1] and Ismael Lares Asseff[2]

[1]Laboratorio de Farmacología, Instituto Nacional de Pediatría, Mexico City, Mexico

[2]Centro Interdisciplinario de Investigación para el Desarrollo Integral Regional (CIIDIR), Instituto Politécnico Nacional, Durango, Mexico

ABSTRACT

The usual therapeutic management of drugs is their application in subsequent doses at different intervals of administration which could be every 6, 8, 12 or 24 hours. However in occasions, their application could be for a prolonged period or for life when they are required to be taken in chronic form as in the case of antihypertensive, antiepileptic and hypoglycemic drugs among others.

The stationary state (ss) of drugs is usually reached after 8 half-lives of elimination for drugs administered for therapeutic purposes. Hence, from the point of view of safety and efficacy, it is convenient that once

* Corresponding author: Gabriela Pérez Guillé, Laboratorio de Farmacología, Instituto Nacional de Pediatría. Avenida Imán # 1, 3er piso, Col Cuicuilco, CP 04530, Mexico D.F, Mexico, e-mail: reparo_gaby@yahoo.com.mx.

the stationary state is reached, such concentrations should be maintained within the therapeutic range that corresponds to each drug. Such concentrations in a stable state (Css) are achieved when the speed of entry of the drug into the organism is equal to the speed of elimination. However, when the speed of entry is higher than the elimination speed, there is a danger that the concentrations overpass the maximum tolerated concentrations and thus risk of toxicity. On the contrary, when the elimination speed of the drug is higher than the entry speed, there is a danger of having a sub-therapeutic concentrations. Therefore, the principal objective is to reach and maintain the concentrations within the therapeutic range, in such a way that from pharmacokinetic point of view, precise concentration (with small variations between the maximum and minimum concentration) and exact concentration (getting to and maintaining the concentrations within the therapeutic range) are achieved.

INTRODUCTION

In recent years, pharmacokinetic studies characterizing the pharmacokinetics of many drugs have increased. Those studies include individuals under different health conditions. Initial studies used different unique doses designed to determine such parameters as biological half-life, the apparent volume of distribution and metabolism of drugs among others, and aimed at establishing if these parameters are or not dose-dependent. Subsequent studies may involve the administration of a number of equal doses at constant intervals to compare drug accumulation model with pattern predicted from single dose studies and determine whether they have inductive or inhibitory effects on drug metabolism. In the course of these studies of single and multiple doses, it is often possible to determine, with varying degrees of accuracy, the relationship between drug concentrations in plasma and the intensity of the pharmacological effect and observe the possible effects of the disease state of this relationship on the pharmacokinetics of the drug. When there is enough information for a given drug, it is possible to explore the usefulness of monitoring concentrations at steady state in plasma (serum or whole blood) of patients who are regularly taking drugs. Therefore, we will mention the factors affecting the determination, control and clinical interpretation of concentrations at a steady state [1].

The most important thing resulting to a therapeutic standpoint is constant administration of multiple doses of a drug at regular intervals to a patient. In other words, chronic administration of a drug to a patient can lead to a gradual increase in drug blood levels which continues until the steady state concentrations are reached. The risk of drug accumulation occurs if the input speed exceeds the rate of elimination [2-4]. And so, drugs with slow elimination rate should obviously have a higher accumulation [5].

The phenomenon of accumulation leading to steady-state concentrations may differ depending on if the pharmacokinetics are linear or nonlinear.

On considering the steady state levels of drugs with linear pharmacokinetics, the particular drug compartment model or route of administration should be taken into account. Table 1 shows the comparatively short formulas to calculate the concentrations at steady state. For example, when the administration is by intravenous infusion at a constant rate (R), the concentration gradually increases until the input speed (R) is equal to the elimination rate, that is (Kel x Vd) = (CLt). The concentrations at a steady state (Css) or the plateau reached will then correspond to the volume of distribution [6]. If the doses are administered by oral, parenteral or other means at regular intervals (t) then, Css will be equal to FD/Vd x Kel x t, where F is the fraction of the absorbed dose [7]. The average Css calculated from the area under the curve of concentrations at steady state is a function of time of the dosing interval.

It can be seen that the formulas for Css for single or multi-compartment models are very similar. The main difference lies in obtaining Kel and other parameters derived from the terminal slope of the curve of log plasma concentrations versus time (slope = $-\beta/2.303$) and V x β distribution corresponds to the volume defined by Gibaldi et al. [8].

The equations of the average Css for both mono and multi-compartment models show that Css is inversely proportional to Kel and β, given that the biological half-life ($t^{1/2}$) of a drug is 0.693/Kel or $0.693/\beta$, then, Css is proportional to the half-life ($t^{1/2}\beta$). Changes in t ½ β determined by induction or inhibition of drug-metabolizing enzymes or changes in renal function are consequently reflected in changes in Css.

Table 1. Formulas for calculating the concentrations at steady state

Adm. Route	Mono-compart Model	Multi-compart Model
Infusion I.V	Css = R/Kel x Vd	C = R/Vβ x β
Oral route or parenteral routes	Css = FD/Vd x Kel x t	C = FD/V β x (β x t)
Independent route of administration	Area = Css x t	Area = FD/Vβ x β

Css is a comparative indicator of bioavailability due to their proportionality to the fraction of the absorbed dose F. This characteristic has been used to detect and evaluate changes in bioavailability, or differences resulting from changes in the pharmaceutical formulation [9-10]. There are some practical problems for the accurate determination of Css. Given that the steady state concentrations ranging between each dosing interval determined by the effects of absorption, distribution and elimination also show greater fluctuations in the extent the intervals of administration outweigh the t½β. It is therefore better to determine the area under the curve of concentration versus time during a dosing interval, rather than the drug concentration at any time within this range, since a single determination may have variable results, particularly if the drug shows multi-compartment characteristics.

Regular administration of a dose in a dosing interval at a time t of elimination half-life (t½β), determines an average level of concentration corresponding to 1.44 times (FD) which is the absorbed fraction of the dose administered. Thus, the time required for the drug to reach average level of Css or the average amount of drug in the body during steady state (ss) [11, 12], is at least 4 times the half-life, with the drug being independent of t [13.] Thus the degree of accumulation of a drug with linear pharmacokinetics can be defined in terms of the rate of accumulation.

$$\frac{1.44t_{1/2}}{\tau} = \frac{1}{Kel*\tau} = \qquad \text{Equation 1}$$

Sometimes it is difficult or impossible to observe the terminal exponential phase corresponding to the elimination of a drug, particularly when concentrations have decreased by two or more orders of magnitude after administration of a single dose. It is possible under these circumstances to reach a state of apparent plasma equilibrium whereas concentrations of the drug in an organ or tissue acting as a deep compartment continue to increase [14]. This masked accumulation may explain the onset of a delay in the pharmacological effect and that the increase in the strength of pharmacological effect is gradual in time when drug concentrations in plasma appear to be at steady state if the site of action is in the deep compartment.

When pharmacokinetic processes cannot be described by first order kinetics but with a Michaellis Menten kinetics, the pharmacokinetics differ significantly for drugs described by linear elimination kinetics. Some drugs have a pronounced nonlinear behavior or the pharmacokinetics are dose-dependent. This is possibly due to different reasons such as saturation in intestinal transport systems, renal or changes in the binding capacity of the drug protein, the drug effects on organ perfusion or urine pH and flow rate etc. [15]. The most important reason for the nonlinearity is probably the limited capacity of some metabolizing enzyme systems of drugs which involve processes that have to be described by the kinetics of Michaellis Menten because the drug concentrations at the site of biotransformation are not much lower than Michaellis' constant for these processes.

In these circumstances, a re-arrangement of equation is necessary (Equation 2).

$$\bar{C}\infty = \frac{f}{Vd*_{\iota}}$$ Equation 2

This is applicable to the following relationship when it is linear kinetics for a compartment model(Equation 2).

$$\frac{\bar{c}}{fD} = Vd * Ke$$ Equation 3

Which shows that the proportion of the drug concentration at steady state between doses is dose-dependent for drugs with characteristics corresponding to linear pharmacokinetics. On the contrary, this ratio would increase with increasing dose if the removal involves a process of limited capacity [16]. In these circumstances, Css increases proportionally with increasing dose. If a drug is removed only by a route with limited capacity, there will be an unlimited accumulation when F x D/t>Vmax. In these cases, the accumulation of drugs with Michaellis kinetics is dose-dependent and so, the time required to reach concentrations in the steady state will increase with increasing dose and the removal rate will relatively decrease with increasing dose.

Clinical Interpretation of the Levels in the Steady State

The clinical interpretation of drug levels in the steady state can be altered by the presence of pharmacologically active metabolites or by changes in the distribution of the drug that can result in a change in the ratio between the drug plasma concentration and the intensity of the pharmacological effect. A change in the rate of elimination from the central compartment determined by causes such as induction or enzyme inhibition and impaired renal function, can have a pronounced effect on the ratio of drug concentrations in the central and peripheral compartments. The proportion of drug concentrations in both the central compartment and the peripheral differs during the infusion or absorption and distribution phase in the post elimination phase [13] or in the elimination phase [17]. Studies in experimental animals show a marked variation in drug elimination accompanied by changes in drug distribution in the organ in which there is an affectation of the plasma and the biotransformation [18].

All these factors alone cannot completely interpret concentrations at a steady state. Appropriate clinical evaluation of the patient is needed. The determinations of the concentrations at steady state would never replace clinical evaluation. Both form the integral and comprehensive therapeutic assessment tools which are very useful and necessary for the safe and effective design of individualized treatment regimens to assess the bioavailability and patient compliance, as well as to prevent and control drug interactions.

REFERENCES

[1] Levy, G.: Pharmacokinetics monitoring and clinical interpretation of steady-state blood level of drugs. *Clin Pharm Ther*16: 130- 134.1974.

[2] Dost FH. Blood Levels. Kinetics of concentration processes In: The sistemic circulation. Georg Thieme, Leipzjg, 1953.

[3] Wagner, JG, Northam, JI, Alway, CD, and Carpenter, OS, *Nature*, 207: 1301 (1965).

[4] Wilegand, RG, Buddenhagen, JD, and Endicott, CJ, *J. Pharm. Scl.* 52: 268, 1963.

[5] Ausberger, A., Lin Wochschr., 32: 945, 1954.

[6] Dost FH. Fundamentals of pharmacokinetics. Stuttgart, 1968, Georg Thieme Verlag.

[7] Wagner, JG, Northham, JI, Alway, CD, and Carpenter, OS: Blood levels of drug at the equilibrium state after multiple dosing, *Nature*, 207: 1301 to 1302.1965.

[8] Gibaldi, M., Nagashima, R., and Levy, G.: Relationship Between drug concentration in plasma or serum and amount of drug in the body. *J Pharm Sci*58: 193-197, 1969.

[9] Mannlnnen, V., Melin, J., and Hartel, G.: Serum-digoxin treatment With Different Concentrations During preparations, *Lancet,* 2: 934-935, 1971.

[10] Bochner, F., Hooper WD, Tyver, JM, and Eadle, MJ: Factors Involved in an outbreak of phenytoin intoxication, *J Neurol Sci.* 16: 481 to 487.1972.

[11] Van Rossum, JM, and Tomey, AHM: Multicompartment kinetics and the accumulation plateu, *Arch IntPharmacodynTher*188: 200- 203, 1970.

[12] Wagner, JG, Northam, JI, Alway, CD, and Carpenter, O. S: Blood levels of drug at the equilibrium state after multiple dosing. *nature.* 207: 1301 to 1302.1965.

[13] Van Rossum WYD and Tomey, AHM: Rate of accumulation and plateau plasma concentration of drugs after chronic medication, *J Pharm Pharmacol* 20: 390 to 392.1968.

[14] Gibaldi, M. Levy, G., and Weintraub, H.: Drug distribution and pharmacologic effects. *CllnPharmacolTher*12: 734 to 742.1971.

[15] Levy. G.: Dose dependent effect in pharmacoklnetics. In Tedeschi, DH and Tedeschl, RE Editors: Importance of basic principles in drug evaluation, New York, 1968, Raven Press, pp.141-172.

[16] Tsuchiya. F. and Levy. G.: Relationship Between dose and plateau levels of drugs eleminated by parallel first order kinetics and limited capacity. *J Pharm Sci*61: 541-544. 1972.

[17] Gibaldi M: Effect of mode of administration on drug distribution in a two-compartment open system. *J. Pharm. Scl.*58: 327-331.1963.

[18] Jahnchen, E., and Levy, G.: Relationship Between elimination distribution, and anticoagulant action of dicumarol. *J PharmacolExpTher* 188: 293-299, 1974.

In: Optimization of Drug Prescribing in Elderly ISBN: 978-1-63484-879-4
Editors: Juárez O. H. and Lares A. I.

Chapter 9

THE INFLUENCE OF OLDNESS ON PHARMACOKINETICS AND DRUG DISPOSITION

Hugo Juárez Olguín[1,*], Radames Alemon Medina[2] and Ismael Lares Asseff[3]

[1]Laboratorio de Farmacología, Instituto Nacional de Pediatría, Mexico City, Mexico
Departamento de Farmacología, Facultad de Medicina, Universidad Nacional Autónoma de Mexico, Mexico D.F., Mexico
[2]Laboratorio de Farmacología, Instituto Nacional de Pediatría, Mexico City, Mexico
[3]Centro Interdisciplinario de Investigación para el Desarrollo Integral Regional (CIIDIR), Instituto Politécnico Nacional, Durango, México

ABSTRACT

Growth, development and aging form part of a continuous dynamic process that is accompanied by biological, physiological, chemical and mental changes that define the peculiar characteristics in every biological age.

---

[*]Corresponding author: Hugo Juárez Olguín, Laboratorio de Farmacología, Instituto Nacional de Pediatría. Avenida Imán # 1, 3er piso, Col Cuicuilco, CP 04530, Mexico D.F, Mexico. E-mail: juarezol@yahoo.com.

As the chronological age progresses, the development and presentation of sicknesses peculiar to every age range begin to surface. However, the common feature in the aging process is the declining tendency in the physical, mental and functional capacities of the people. All these biological, physiological, chemical and physiopathological changes are accompanied by nutritional disorders which concomitantly would determine important pharmacokinetic and pharmacodynamic changes which in turn would define the peculiar pharmacokinetic characteristics during the aging process. These aspects would influence in the response to treatment as well as in the susceptibility to present drug adverse events.

Introduction

Aging, in the life of the human, is a stage characterized by a series of anatomical and physiological changes. These changes, per se, do not necessarily mean senility but involve pathological conditions that usually lead to a decrease in physical and physiological capacities which are not often considered when nutrients are supplied. In extreme situations, the later may be insufficient for or exceed physiological capacities. The usual requirement of nutrients and micronutrients at younger ages normally witnesses some kind of modification as growth and development take place and this modification depends on multiple causes and age [1].

Drug administration in elderly people most often do not take into account the above aspects, a situation which frequently leads to therapeutic failure and/ or drug toxicity. In addition to the changes typical of aging, old age is characterized by a higher incidence of diseases that increase with age, and hence condition a therapeutic approach with a greater number of drugs that are simultaneously used which gives way to a higher probability of drug interactions.

These issues have compelled us to search for methods that would better explain the pharmacokinetics of drugs and their understanding in order to make more rational therapeutic management of drugs in elderly patients.

Absorption

A number of physiological changes in the gastrointestinal (GI) tract take place as people get older. Among such changes are some esophageal defects as dilation, relaxation of the lower sphincter, impaired esophageal emptying, and increased non-expulsive contractions that provoke swallowing defects [1] and hence alter the absorption of drugs. Therefore, it is necessary to consider these changes when a drug is being prescribed to avoid dosage forms that are difficult to swallow. In Table 1, age related GI physiological changes affecting absorption are shown.

Table 1. Age related physiological changes that can affect drug absorption [1-9, 13]

Mouth:
– Loss of teeth.
– Decreased salivary secretion.
Esophagus:
– Dilatation.
– Relaxation of the lower sphincter.
– Delay in esophageal emptying.
– Increase in non-expulsive contractions.
Stomach:
– Decreased acid secretion.
– Increase in the pH.
– Decreased splenic blood flow.
– Decline of gastric emptying time.
– Decline of the surface area of tissue.
Bowel:
– Atrophy of the mucosa.
– Proliferation of connective tissue.
– Sclerotic fibrous tissue formation.
– Atrophy of the crypts.
– Increased amyloid in submucosa.
– Decline in the number of enterocytes.
– Decrease in Peyer's patches.
– Thickening of the muscles of the colon.
– Active uptake is decreased for some substances (iron, thiamine, etc.).
– Reduction in the intestinal perfusion.

The effect of age at gastric level is a decrease of acid secretion. This activity decreases by 25-35% when compared with its production at 20 years old. Moreover, the gastric pH also increases with age [1, 2], and thus prejudices he ionization and solubility of many drugs. In addition, the splenic blood flow, [1, 3] is found to decrease with age and in line with this is a reduction in the gastric emptying time and its tissue surface area [2, 3]. Although the stomach is not directly involved in drug absorption, the gastric pH facilitates the solubility of some drugs and so, improves their entry into the portal blood stream [4].

In small bowel like in rats, changes that are characterized by proliferation of connective tissue and formation of fibrous tunic sclera have been reported. [5] As a function of increasing age, it is also found that the crypts come to be widely separated and that there is a higher incidence of atrophy; an increase in the amyloid content of the sub-mucosa and a decline in the number of enterocytes [5, 6]. Moreover, there is a decrease in the number of Peyer's patches and follicles within them while the muscles of the colon becomes thickened [7]. The passive absorption, mediated by the entry of xylose is reduced, but this is only significant in elderly people from 80 years and above. For most drugs, the speed or the extent of absorption are not altered as a result of physiological changes in the aging of the gastrointestinal tract, although this is still controversial [8, 9]. With advancing age, active absorption processes are reported to be significantly decreased, based on the unlimited absorption found for iron, calcium, galactose, thiamine, vitamin B12 and 3-methyl glucose.

Presently, there are few studies that take into account the absorption of medications in elderly patients. Digoxin [10] and chlordiazepoxide [11] have been reported to have a slight delay in absorption. In a study of Varoquaux O. et al., in elderly people, it was found that the pharmacokinetics of trimethoprim and sulfametoxazole were altered [12].

Reduction of intestinal perfusion may decrease the absorption of some drugs, especially those that are highly soluble in lipids. The concentration gradient of the drug that crosses the serosal surface declines as a result of reduction in the flow rate. Furthermore, at about 65 years of age, the cardiac output decreases by 30% leading to a decrease of 45% to 50% of blood flow to the gastrointestinal tract as well as in the liver and kidneys. Although many physiological changes occur in the gastrointestinal tract in individuals over 65 years, very few changes occur in the absorption of drugs [13].

Table 2. Age related physiological changes affecting drug distribution in the elderly [14-18]

Changes in Body Composition:
– Decreased total body water.
– Decreased intracellular water.
– Decreased lean body mass.
Changes in drug Union and Tissue Plasma Protein:
– Decreased concentration of serum albumin.
– Increased acid glycoprotein concentrations.
– Changes in the number of binding sites.
– Changes in the constant of affinity.
Circulatory changes and organ perfusion:
– Decreased cardiac output.
– Increase in sympathetic tone.
– Increase in peripheral resistance.
– Change in tissue permeability.

In a research conducted with intramuscularly administered drugs in older individuals, it was observed that the rate of absorption decreased. This phenomenon of slow absorption could probably be attributed to lower activity in the elderly [6].

DISTRIBUTION

There are some factors which can influence the volume of distribution of drugs in the elderly. Among these factors are those impacting on body composition, which determine the particular characteristics of each age along the processes of growth, development and aging, and could modify the distribution of certain compounds [14]. In Table 2, these age related factors affect drug distribution in the elderly are summarized.

Metabolically active tissues are gradually and slowly replaced with age. From 15 to 60 years old, body fat increases from 18-36% in men and 33-48% in women. As a result, there is a reduction in lean body mass to body weight ratio. Hence, drugs that are mainly liposoluble should have a higher volume of distribution in women than in men, while for drugs that are highly hydrosoluble, the plasma concentrations are higher in view of the decrease volume of distribution. On the other part, total body water decreases by approximately 10-15% in the period from 20 to 85 years of age, while the extracellular water remains almost unchanged with reductions of approximately 0.37 for men and 0.27% for women. The intracellular water is reduced from 42% at 25 years to 35% at 73 years of age. Given that the lean body mass is reduced per unit of body weight in the elderly, drugs that are primarily distributed in lean body mass will exhibit higher plasma levels compared to young adults. In the absence of binding of antipyrine to albumin, the body water which declines with age should form the apparent volume of distribution [15, 16]. For other drugs, the apparent volume of distribution penetrates extravascular tissues.

Studies have shown that albumin concentrations decrease with age, while the concentrations of gamma globulin increase. These changes are attributable to the relative inactivity in most elderly patients. This decrease in albumin will result in reduced sites for drugs that mainly bound to it. Therefore, the administration of several drugs in elderly people may lead to competition for the few existing binding sites, which for many drugs are similar, in such a way that there is a shift in the binding site of one drug to another site of attachment and this would change the distribution of the drugs [17].

More recently, interest has increased on drug bindings to other blood components such as erythrocytes and 1-acid glycoprotein (AGP) which are the binding sites for basic drugs (cations) including chlorpromazine and primaquine [18]. Recently, an increases in the acute phase reactant (acid 1glicoproteína) in relation to age was demonstrated [19].

The distribution of drugs may also be altered by variations in the rate and amount of blood flow in different organs. As a compensatory phenomenon to the decreased cardiac output, there is an increase in sympathetic tone, permitting preferential blood flow to the vital organs with a concomitant decrease in renal flow and peripheral blood [20]. There is a decrease in liver blood flow of approximately 0.3 to 1.5% per year after 20 years, partly explained by the decrease in cardiac output. With aging, there is a hardening of the arteries by arteriosclerosis characterized by the deposit of cholesterol in arterial walls and a decrease in blood vessel elastin [21].

Changes in the volume of distribution may change the time of elimination half-life ($t_{1/2el}$) and, when the distribution volume increases, the elimination half-life also increases. It has been suggested that bed rest may have an indirect effect on the distribution of the drug. The degree of physical activity is a possible mechanism that contributes to certain pharmacokinetic alterations in senescent individuals. Variations in permeability in tissues are other reasons given to explain changes in drug distribution in the elderly [22].

METABOLISM

The ability of biotransformation and/or biodegradation of a substance introduced in the body enables the substance to be removed after a series of biochemical transformations that change the substance into a more polar and a less soluble compound (metabolite) different from the unchanged molecule and in this form, the excretion is increased and the volume of distribution is decreased. Biotransformation does not only favor the removal of drugs but also often produces inactivation compound. Although sometimes, some metabolites have pharmacological activity [23].

The capacity of an organ (liver, kidney, etc.) to eliminate or clear a drug from the blood depends on the balance of the following three factors [24]:

a) Blood flow to the organ.
b) The inherent capacity of the drug to metabolize or be secreted (intrinsic clearance).
c) The binding to blood components.

The most important organ involved in metabolism is the liver. Hepatic metabolism of drugs can activate a drug, finish its pharmacological action and/or generate a polar ionized metabolite which is easily excreted by the kidney.

The liver cells change with age. The weight decreases by 1.6% to 2.5% of the body weight while after 30 years of life, its irrigation begins to decline by 0.3 to 1.5% every year and at 65, the reduction in blood flow is approximatcly 40% [25]. Although routine liver function test do not change with age, this fact docs not reflect a loss of the capacity in hepatic metabolism of drugs. Changes in blood flow to the liver alter the steady state levels of intravenously administered drugs and affect first step removal (Table 3).

Delayed clearance of indocyanine green, a compound highly extracted by the liver seems to reflect the decline of blood flow to the liver with age. As previously noted, the decrease in cardiac output from 30 to 40% at 65 years of age, brings about a reduction of blood flow to the liver by about 12 to 40%. If hepatic metabolism is maintained, this reduction in hepatic blood flow could result in a decrease in extraction of highly clarified drug (e.g., hepatic extraction ratio is 0.70), as was confirmed for propranolol [26, 27].

The body has many nonspecific enzymes that catalyze a variety of reactions that ultimately lead to the formation of a variety of metabolites. Many years ago, Williams et al. reported that most of the reactions occurring during drug metabolism can be classified into two general phases [28]. The first phase comprises of all the reactions that convert one functional group into another (e.g., oxidation of alcohol to acetaldehyde and acetic acid), decomposition of neutral compounds to fragments having polar groups (e.g., hydrolysis include ethers and amides) or introduction of polar groups into non-polar compounds (e.g., hydroxylation of aliphatic and aromatic components). The second phase includes all the reactions that combine polar groups of compounds (Table 4).

Recent studies of the nature of these oxidative systems showed that most of the enzymes require NADPH as much as oxygen [29]. Recently, it was shown that these reactions are catalyzed by a number of heme proteins known as cytochrome p 450 [30].

There are varieties of reactions catalyzed by various cytochrome P-450 in liver microsomes. As a result of the reactions of the different enzymes of cytochrome P450, a specific compound usually undergoes, in simultaneous form, various reactions that convert it into different metabolites. A drug can be converted into a number of different metabolites by a variety of reactions and each can be catalyzed by different enzymes [31].

There are a number of evidences indicating a decline of MFOS in age-related liver, and in clinical studies, it was found that the elimination time of drugs in the elderly is more prolonged. In nutshell, the results of these studies suggest that the reactions of Phase I undergo age-dependent decline, while Phase II reactions or conjugations seem not to be affected.

Table 3. Age-related physiological changes affecting drug metabolism [20-45]

In liver:
Anatomical alterations:
– Decreased weight (mass). Circulatory disorders.
– Decreased blood flow. Metabolic (or enzyme) changes.
– Decreased reactions. Phase I oxidative functions are diminished due to:
a) Loss of microsomal membrane and/or MFOS (mixed function oxidase system) constituents.
b) Decrease in the quality of the enzyme and the MFOS hemoproteins.
c) MFOS generated microsomal changes.
d) Decrease in inducible oxidative functions.
– Decrease in the activities of enzymes induced by MFOS.
– Decrease in the speed and extent of MFOS induction by medication.
– Decrease in the total enzyme activity with increasing age.

Table 4. Classification of general reactions during drug metabolism proposed by Williams [28]

Phase 1 reactions: General route of drug metabolism
– Oxidation reactions
– NADPH-dependent oxygenases mixed in liver microsomes. Dehydrogenation: Alcohols aldehyde oxidase (monoamine oxidase).
– Reduction Reactions
– Azoreduction Microsomes.
– Nitroreduction Microsomes.
– Carbonylreduction.
– Hydrolysis reactions
– De-esterification.
– De-amination.
Phase 2 reactions
– Formation of glucuronide. Metilation.
– Acylation: acetate, amino acids.
– Formation of mercapturic acid. Sulphate Conjugate.
– Formation of dihydrodial.

The classical studies of Kato et al. [32] demonstrated a direct correlation between chronological age and liver MFOS enzymes´ activities. The results of these and subsequent studies have shown age-dependent decline in the enzymatic activities. The first of this decline is seen in *in-vivo* and *in-vitro* metabolisms of various drugs. The second is the absence of induction of MFOS enzymes and the third is a decline in the rate and extent of drug induction of MFOS.

A well documented age-dependent decline is in the function of liver MFOS microsomes attributed to:

1) A loss of the microsomal membrane and/or MFOS constituents.
2) Decline in the quality of the enzymes and hemoproteins of MFOS.
3) Changes in the middle of microsomal MFOS, or
4) Combinations of the above among others [33].

The effect of aging on the oxidative metabolism of drugs is also complicated by smoking habits. Clearance is more pronounced in smokers as demonstrated in studies carried out with oral antipyrine and propranolol [34]. In some cases, the declining function of MFOS reflects a decreased use of common enzyme inducers (cigarettes, alcohol, certain foods) in the elderly [35]. Cederbaum et al. [36] noted that in the elderly, poor nutrition is the least of the three things that is partly responsible for the decline of the microsomal enzyme function. They noted that both vitamin C and folate are often below the therapeutic levels in the elderly. In humans, the effect of aging on glucuronide conjugation has not been well understood, since a number of drugs can be administered orally or intravenously. However, Greenblatt et al. [37], demonstrated with lorazepam, that although glucuronidation appeared to decline with age, this decline was not statistically significant when cigarette smokers were omitted from the analysis of the data. In contrast to the changes noted for oxidative route conjugation reactions, in phase II, as already noted, these reactions appear to be intact in the elderly. The acetylation seems to be affected with aging [38].

Studies in rats have shown that the actions of pentobarbital, secobarbital and other drugs that are presumably metabolized by liver cytochrome P-450 are more elongated in seminal animals than in younger animals. In a series of articles, Kato et al. [39] reported that a more prolonged effect of drugs is determined by an increase in biological half-life due to a decrease in the ability of the liver to metabolize such drugs. In rats, the decline in overall enzyme activity increases with age, however, this was not only due to a decrease in the amount of cytochrome P 450, cytochrome C reductase activity and NADPH per gram of liver but also for the decrease in the weight of the liver [39, 40].

The activity of non-microsomal enzymes can also change with age. Jha and Rizvi [41] reported a decline in cholinesterase activity with age in men when acetylcholine or succinylcholine were used as substrates, whereas no changes were observed in women. Another important non-microsomal route for drug metabolism involves acetylation. A study with isoniazid, which undergoes hepatic acetylation, showed no difference in clearance rates among young subjects (10-24 years) and older ones (over 65 years). This suggests that acetylation is not significantly affected by aging [42]. Ethanol is also affected by the liver alcohol cytosolic dehydrogenase. Though a microsomal component, ethanol oxidation system (MEOS) contributes by 20 to 25% in the processes of acetylation depending on the plasma concentrations of the drug. Most data support that the elderly are less able to metabolize ethanol than young people and as a result suffer a higher incidence of ethanol toxicity [43].

The effects of age on the biliary excretion has been little explored. However, a decrease in liver function and blood flow to the organ in the elderly, it is inevitable that the biliary clearance would decrease. Certain compounds including cardiac glycoside ouabain, are probably faster and actively excreted into the bile in the absence of any biotransformation in the liver. Transport of drugs and other compounds from the plasma, through the hepatocyte into the bile space is another feature that may be affected with increasing age [44, 45].

Although drugs are metabolized by a variety of enzymes, however, the descriptions obtained with a drug should not be extrapolated to other drugs. The metabolism of one drug is frequently different from another. It should be emphasized that the activities of many enzymes that metabolize drugs may be altered by the state of disease, diet and substances that are not nutrients as well as the environment [43-45]. Because the habit of the elderly are constantly changing and that they are more susceptible to more diseases, which generally result in different degrees of irreversible changes in some organs containing enzymes that metabolize drugs, it is difficult to distinguish intrinsic changes of drug clearance caused by these factors and those directly caused by the processes of aging. It is important to mention that the elimination half-lives of drugs in the elderly as well as the hepatic metabolism have an important variability [44-46]. However, changes in the metabolism itself is reflected through the clearance. An example is diazepam, where the increase in the elimination half-life is in proportion to changes in the volume of distribution with age and which does not reflection altered metabolism [47, 48].

In chronic treatment, the plasma concentrations accumulate at a rate dependent on the elimination half-life, but concentrations in steady state depends on the clearance steady state. The result of these is that when the elimination half-life is increased and the clearance is not modified, the steady state concentrations are slowly reached and fluctuations between the minimum and maximum plasma concentrations are higher but the average concentration remains the same. Although most studies suggest an age-dependent decline in the activities as well as the adaptive capacity of hepatic microsomal drug metabolizing enzymes, we must be careful in interpreting such suggestion since most experimental work do not necessarily reflect what happens in the human body [49].

Renal Excretion

For a great number of unchanged drugs and/or metabolites that are biotransformed into less toxic products, the kidney is the main organ of their excretion. Thus, the anatomophysilogical changes of the kidney as a result of increasing age, will affect the ability to excrete a drug and/or its metabolites.

Renal excretion of drugs and/or its metabolites is a result of filtration, secretion and tubular resorption, as well as pH, blood flow to the kidney and urinary flow.

From the anatomical point of view, in the period from 20 to 80 years of age, there is a decrease of 20% in the size of the kidneys and this will invariably reduce the glomerular filtration. In addition, there is a loss of 35% in the number of functional glomeruli and 30% in the number of nephrons. Moreover, the renal blood flow is found to reduce by 45 to 53%. The consequence of all these changes is a reduction in creatinine clearance which declines each year by 0.5-1.0 ml/min in healthy elderly people. In nutshell, all these result in a loss of approximately 50% of renal function in individuals above 85 years of age. The increase in serum creatinine is due to decreased glomerular filtration and tubular secretion [50].

Since lean body mass declines with age, the production of endogenous creatinine also decreases as age increases. So, creatinine clearance tends to fall significantly in the elderly before the serum creatinine increases. Therefore, the serum creatinine may be normal in the elderly while renal function is substantially reduced. This entails the calculation of creatinine through nomograms in the elderly people [51].

Tubular reabsorption plays an important role in the excretion of drugs. This action depends on the size of molecules excreted, the concentration gradient in the tubules, lipid solubility properties of the molecules and finally, the pH of the tubular filter [50, 51].

As a consequence of aging, there are some changes at renal tubular level that may or may not affect both the extent and the rate of absorption of the drug molecules. The way the absorption rate and its extent is affected is outlined below [51-53].

1) There is a decreased ability to concentrate the water coming into the renal tubules after glomerular filtration.
2) There is a reduction in the capacity of reabsorption of sodium and phosphorous.
3) Aging reduces the acidity gradient and hence brings about a decrease in the ability to acidify the urine.

There are a number of drugs and/or its metabolites excreted by the kidneys. And taking into considerations of the changes which these organs undergo along the time, therapeutic management in older patients should require adequate knowledge of these changes. Also it should be born in mind that these changes could be modified by disease states and/or drug interactions.

REFERENCES

[1] Schmucker DL. Drug disposition in the elderly: a review of critical factors. *J. Am. Geriatr Soc.*1984;32(2):144-149.

[2] Ritschel W. Disposition of drugs in geriatric patients. *Pharm. Int.*1980; 1:226-230.

[3] Greenblatt DJ, Von Moltke LL, Harmatz JS et al. Pharmacokinetics, pharmacodynamics, and drug disposition. In: Davis KL, Charney D, Coyle JT et al., eds. *Neuropsychopharmacology: The Fifth Generation of Progress*. 5th ed. Philadelphia: Lippincott Williams and Wilkins; 2002:507-524.

[4] Pénzes L, Salmon G, Winter M. Intestinal absorption and utilization of radiomethionine in old age. *Exp. Gerontol.* 1968: 257-63.

[5] Pénzes L. Further data on the age dependent intestinal absorption of dibasic amino acids. *ExpGerontol.* 1974; 9 (5-6): 259-262.

[6] Lascalea MC. The digestive system in old age. *Excerpta Med Z.* 1959; 2: 419-422.

[7] Hoshi H, Horie K, Tanaka K, Nagata H et al. Patterns of age-dependent changes in the numbers of lymphfollicles and germinal centres in somatic and mesenteric lymphnodes in growing C57Bl/6 mice. *J Anat.* 2001; 198(Pt 2): 189-205.

[8] Wooten JM. Pharmacotherapy Considerations in Elderly Adult. *South. Med. J.* 2012;105(8):437-445.

[9] Andrew W, Benke RH, Shimlzu Y. Variations in cell population intestinal lamina propria in relation to age. *Geront.* 1966; 12:129-143.

[10] Chen R, Zou SL, Wang ML et al. Population pharmacokinetics of digoxin in elderly patients. *Eur J Drug Metab Pharmacokinet.* 2013;38 (2):115-21.

[11] Greenblatt DJ, Divoll MK, Abernethy DR et al. Age and gender effects on chlordiazepoxide kinetics: relation to antipyrine disposition. *Pharmacology.* 1989;38(5):327-34.

[12] Varoquaux O, Lajoie D, Gobert C et al. Pharmacokinetics of the trimethoprim-sulphamethoxazole combination in the elderly. *Br. J. Clin. Pharmacol.* 1985;20(6):575-81.

[13] D'Souza AL. Ageing and the gut. *Post. Grad. Med J.* 2007; 83(975): 44-53.

[14] Ueda K, Omae T, Fujishima M. Physiological and biochemical changes in age in based on a population survey in a Japanese community. Hisayama. *Ann. Acad. Med. Singapore*. 1987;16(1):35-41.

[15] Going S, Williams D, Lohman T. Aging and body composition: biological changes and methodological issues. *Exerc. Sport. Sci. Rev.* 1995;23:411-58.

[16] Abbatecola A, Windham BG, Bandinell S et al. Clinical and Biochemical Evaluation Changes Over Aging. Chapter 7. Biological Basis of Geriatric Oncology. *Volume 124 of the series Cancer Treatment and Research.* pp. 135-162.

[17] Silawat N, Savalia, JK, Patel D. Comparative study of impact of age in physiological variables, body composition and blood cholesterol in selected physical education professionals. *Jour. Exer. Scie. and Phys.* 2009; 5 (1): 62-66.

[18] Kennedy E, Frischer H. Distribution of primaquine in human blood: drug-binding to alpha 1-glycoprotein. *J. Lab. Clin. Med.* 1990;116(6): 871-8.

[19] Uysal A, Roach CH. Acute phase reactants. *Acta Medica* 2013; 2: 2-7.

[20] Wooten JM. Pharmacotherapy considerations in elderly adults. *South. Med. J.* 2012;105(8):437-445.

[21] McLean AJ, Le Couteur DG. Aging biology and geriatric clinical pharmacology. *Pharmacol. Rev*. 2004;56:163-184.

[22] Crooks J, O'Malley K, Stevenson IH. Pharmacokinetics in the elderly. *Clin. Pharmacokinet*. 1976;1(4):280-96.

[23] Klotz U. Pharmacokinetics and drug metabolism in the elderly. *Drug. Metab. Rev.* 2009; 41(2):67-76.

[24] Toutain PI, Bousquet ME. Plasma clearance. *J. Vet. Pharmacol. Ther*. 2004;27: 415-425.

[25] Mangoni A.A, Jackson SHD. Age-related changes in pharmacokinetics and pharmacodynamics: basic principles and practical applications. *Br. J. Clin. Pharmacol.* 2004; 57(1): 6-14.

[26] Christian E, Kerstin A., Brigitte V. Regulation of hepatic blood flow: The hepatic arterial buffer response revisited. *World. J. Gastroenterol.* 2010; 16(48): 6046-6057.

[27] Allan J. Mc Lean, David G. Le Couteur. Aging biology and geriatric clinical pharmacology. *Pharmacol. Rev*. 2004; 56:163-184.

[28] Williams RT. *Detoxication mechanisms.* 2nd Edition. John Wiley and Sons: New York, 1959, p. 796.

[29] David L. NOX enzymes and the biology of reactive oxygen. *Nature Reviews Immunology* 2004;4: 181-189.

[30] Mansuy D. Cytochromes P-450 and model systems: great diversity of catalyzed reactions. *Pureand Appl. Chem.* 1994; 66(4): 737-744.

[31] Guengerich FP and Munro AW. Unusual cytochrome P450 enzymes and reactions. *J. Biol. Chem.* 2013; 288 (24): 17065-17073.

[32] Kato R, Takanaka A. Effect of phenobarbital on electron transport system, oxidation and reduction of drugs in liver microsomes of rats of different age. *J. Biochem.* 1968; 63(3):406-8.

[33] Wauthier V, Verbeeck RK, Buc Calderon P. The effect of ageing on cytochrome P450 enzymes: consequences for drug biotransformation in the elderly. *Curr. Medic. Chem.* 2007; 14:745-757.

[34] Barry M, Feely J. Enzyme induction and inhibition. *Pharmac. Ther.* 1990; 48:71-94.

[35] Hutchison LC, O'Brien CE. Changes in pharmacokinetics and pharmacodynamics in the elderly patient. *J. Pharm. Prac.* 2007;20:4-12.

[36] Cederbaum AI. Molecular mechanisms of the microsomal mixed function oxidases and biological and pathological implications. Re*dox Biol.* 2015; 4: 60-73.

[37] Greenblatt DJ, Harmatz JS, Shader RI. Clinical pharmacokinetics of anxiolytics and hypnotics in the elderly. Therapeutic considerations (part II). *Clin. Pharmacokinet.* 1991b; 21 (4): 262-273.

[38] Jin-Ying Lu, Yu-Yi Lin, Heng Zhu et al. Protein acetylation and aging. *Aging*. 2011; 3(10): 911-912.

[39] Kato R, Gillette JR. Sex differences in the effects of abnormal physiological states on the metabolism of drugs by rat liver microsomes. *J. Pharmacol. Exp. Ther.* 1965; 150(2):285-91.

[40] Kato R, Takayanagi M, Oshima T. Differences in the oxidative metabolism of drugs by liver microsomes. *J. Pharmacol.* 1969;19(1): 53-62.

[41] Jha R, Rizvi SI. Age-dependent decline in erythrocyte acetylcholinesterase activity: correlation with oxidative stress. *Biomed. Pap. Med. Fac.* Univ. Palacky. Olomouc. Czech. Repub. 2009;153(3): 195-8.

[42] Loureiro AI, Fernandes C, Bonifácio MJ et al. N-Acetylation of etamicastat, a reversible dopamine-b-Hydroxylase inhibitor. *Drug. Metab. Dispos.*2013; 41:2081-2086.

[43] Reid MC, Anderson PA. Geriatric substance use disorders. *Med. Clin. North. Am*. 1997; 81(4):999-1016.

[44] Kazuto T, Yukihiro S. Liver physiology and liver diseases in the elderly. *World. J. Gastroenterol*. 2013; 19(46): 8459-8467.

[45] Walter S, Klotz U. Influence of diet and nutritional status on drug metabolism. *Clin. Pharmacokinet*. 1996; 31(1):47-64.

[46] Lin J H, Lu A. Role of pharmacokinetics and metabolism in drug discovery and development. *Pharmacol. Rev*. 1997; 49(4): 403-449.

[47] Bernus I, Dickinson RG, Hooper WD et al. Anticonvulsant therapy in aged patients. clinical pharmacokinetic considerations. *Drugs. Aging*. 1997; 10(4):278-89.

[48] Kamijo Y, Hayashi I, Nishikawa T. Pharmacokinetics of the active metabolites of ethylloflazepate in elderly patients who died of asphyxia associated with benzodiazepine-related toxicity. *J. Anal. Toxicol*. 2005; 29(2):140-4.

[49] Maganti L, Panebianco DL, Maes AL. Evaluation of methods for estimating time to steady state with examples from Phase 1 Studies. *AAPS J*. 2008; 10(1): 141-147.

[50] Weinstein JR. Anderson S. The aging kidney: physiological changes. *Adv. Chronic. Kidney. Dis*. 2010; 17(4): 302-307.

[51] Gerry R. Age-related physiological changes and their clinical significance. *West. J. Med*. 1981; 135(6): 434-440.

[52] Rodriguez D. The aging kidney. *Kidney Int*. 1998; 54: 2247-2265.

[53] Mangoni AA, Jackson SH. Age-related changes in pharmacokinetics and pharmacodynamics: basic principles and practical applications. *Br. J. Clin. Pharmacol*. 2004; 57 (1): 6-14.

In: Optimization of Drug Prescribing in Elderly ISBN: 978-1-63484-879-4
Editors: Juárez O. H. and Lares A. I.

Chapter 10

EFFECT OF OLDNESS ON PHARMACOKINETICS OF ANTIBIOTICS

Ismael Lares Asseff[1,*], Alejandra Toledo López[2] and Diego Zamora de la Cruz[3]

[1]Centro Interdisciplinario de Investigación para el Desarrollo Integral Regional (CIIDIR), Instituto Politécnico Nacional, Durango, México
[2]Laboratorio de Farmacología, Instituto Nacional de Pediatría, Mexico City, Mexico
[3]Departamento de Farmacología, Facultad de Medicina, UniversidadNacional Autónoma de Mexico, Mexico City, Mexico

ABSTRACT

Infectious processes in old-aged people constitute an important factor for morbidity and mortality, and play an important role in epidemiological aspects. As part of aging process, there is a decline in the mechanisms of immunological defense accentuated by problems of disability and concomitant pathologies. In the same way, there are risk factors as hospital infections, living in low resource old-age homes and invasive diagnostic procedures which increase the infections and their gravity. Complications of the infections and development of septicemia

*Corresponding author: Ismael Lares Asseff. Instituto Politécnico Nacional, CIIDIR-Unidad Durango, Calle Sigma 119. Fracc. 20 de noviembre II, Durango. Durango, Mexico, C.P. 34220. E-mail: ismaelares@yahoo.com.

secondary to pneumonic processes, infected pressure ulcers or abdominal infections are usually frequent in old age people. From the clinical point of view, there is a masking of the infectious processes since most often, the absence of fever and elevation of leucocytes even in the case of bacteremia is common and even when symptoms exist, they are normal unspecific and these may lead to difficulty in the diagnosis and timely antibiotic treatment of such infections thereby, putting the life of the patient at risk. On the basis of the above, it is recommended the use of antibiotics of wide spectrum with lesser possibilities of adverse effects in advanced age people. Such management, from all intent and purposes, would require a good knowledge of pharmacokinetic characteristics of the antibiotics and the changes owing to the processes of aging.

INTRODUCTION

Elderly patients are potentially at risk of intoxication when the same dosing regimens used in young adults are applied to them [1, 2]. Lately, a number of studies have considered the use of drugs in the elderly in order to determine their safety and effectiveness [3]. Although, a number of comparisons of pharmacokinetic behavior of some drugs in younger populations and old aged people have been made, it is important and necessary to extend these pharmacokinetic comparative studies to other drugs. Interestingly, concern in explaining these pharmacokinetic differences between these two populations is gradually increasing and attention has been focused on the effects of age on the mechanisms of drugs so as to achieve the effectiveness and efficacy required in the treatment of the diseases of the elderly [3-5].

Early studies carried out by Noreddin et al. [6] described optimal dosing design for antibiotic therapy in the elderly. Leikola and Vartia [7] reported half-life of 0.55 hr for penicillin G for younger population and 1 hour for elderly group. Also, in the case of procaine penicillin clearance, a half-life of approximately 10 hours was found in younger population compared to 18 hours in elderly group. These differences were attributed to reduced tubular secretion of antibiotic due to a decrease in renal function with age by researchers.

Vartia and Leikola [8] extended their work to include dihydrostreptomycin and tetracycline. In these cases, they found that the half-life of dihydrostreptomycin was 5.2 hr in younger people compared with 8.4 hr in aged people. Similar observations was noted with tetracycline with half-lives of 4.5 hr. in the elderly against 3.5 hr. in young adults. Bohr et al. [9] and Simon et al. [10] also made similar observations with other antibiotics.

Infectious Processes in the Elderly

Owing to physiological changes of aging, which are characterized by a decline of some physiological processes [11], the elderly are more prone to infectious diseases and are less able to adequately defend themselves against infections as was reported by Gardner [12]. The arrival of adequate concentrations of antimicrobial agents to sites of infection are required [13]. This may be difficult to achieve due to the increasing decline of the already mentioned physiological processes in the elderly and which may even predispose them to unexpected toxicity, especially when several drugs which can act adversely against a given antibiotic are concomitantly used, or when the adverse effects of aging processes which often are unpredictable affect the actions of the drugs [11].

Immunological Aspects in the Elderly

After 60 years of age there is a greater likelihood of developing various diseases which can compromise the defense mechanism, such as atherosclerosis senescent more susceptible to a variety of infections. A loss of consciousness due to any cause and more likely in elderly people can lead to aspiration problems, and/or lower respiratory tract infections [14].

The elderly often have little mobility and periods of immobility or disabling diseases can predispose bedsores susceptible to infection [15]. Also, as a result of the problems of prostatic hypertrophy, there is a higher incidence of urinary tract infections, or concomitant instrumental procedures that may bring about urinary tract infections.

The ability of the immune response decreases with old age. The number of T cells are found to decrease as the age increase [16] and so, the immunological functions are less responsive.

The function of B cells is also found to be diminished in the elderly [17]. Therefore, these immunological factors strongly influence in the susceptibility of the elderly patients to infections and so predispose them to therapeutic use of antibiotics. Hence, pharmacokinetic studies that would allow us to improve the effectiveness and safety of antibiotics used in individuals over 60 years old [18, 19] are of paramount importance.

PHARMACOLOGICAL, CLINICAL AND BIOLOGICAL ASPECTS FOR ANTIBIOTIC THERAPEUTIC OPTIMIZATION IN GERIATRIC PATIENTS

Aging is a normal process in living things characterized by changes in biological and physiological processes which tend to decrease as the age advances. Prominent among these changes is a decrease in renal function. Invariably, the later would affect, among others, the renal excretion of some antibiotics as aminoglycosides, vancomycin, penicillins and some cephalosporins [20-22]. In the same way, aging is marked by a reduction in the capacity of hepatic biotransformation of drugs and this event affects the elimination of some antibiotics like metronidazole, cephoperazone, cephotaxime, tetracycline, sulfametoxazol, ciprofloxacine, antituberculosis etc. [23-25].

It is important to note that bacterial infections are the most frequent cause of hospital admissions and leads to 30% of death in geriatric population [22]. The infections which the elderly are mostly predisposed are urinary tract infection, pneumonia, infections of the soft tissues and intra-abdominal infections, mainly determined by different microorganisms that require different antibiotics depending on the antimicrobial susceptibility and the infection site.

The urinary tract infections should be seriously considered if they correspond to upper tract, since their treatment requires a prolonged period of time than in lower tract. It is very rare that the treatment of infections due to asymptomatic bacteriuria is well. Soft tissue infections are produced by cellulites and infected ulcer of pressure (of decubitus) due to diabetic foot or peripheral vascular diseases [26]. Infections in the elderly that require long term antibiotic management need special monitoring, since they may be due to organisms resistant to some antibiotics especially in patients that have been previously treated with such drugs.

Important aspects to bear in mind when prescribing antibiotics in the elderly are the side effects and their timely detection through pharmacovigilance. In some occasions, it is difficult to know which drug was the causal agent of the side effects since polypharmacy is frequently common in this group of patients for the high necessity of various drugs for the treatment of concomitant sicknesses like diabetes and arterial hypertension [27].

The design of optimum dosage regimens for antimicrobial therapy in the elderly should take into account the following: advance aged people frequently present concomitantly repeated infections in combination with other sicknesses as cardiovascular disorders, metabolic diseases or malignant diseases which need antibiotic treatment due to added infectious processes and thus, there is an increased risk of polypharmacy and potential risk of drug interactions and/or pharmacodynamics [6].

The increase in the population of advance aged people in all the world represents a great challenge since this means an increase in the cases of infectious disease peculiar to this age. Consequently, we are compelled to search for and develop better antibiotics and therapeutic schemes that would cover the spectra of infections presented in the elderly and bearing in mind that some of them could be resistant to some of these drugs. However, there are always benefits as well as risks of toxic effects and unfavorable interactions with other drugs. Based on the above, it is essential to optimize therapeutic management in these patients using the pharmacodynamic principles with peculiar characteristics of aging. Invariably, this would help in reducing bacterial resistance and the toxic effects of antibiotics [28].

It is important to consider the incapacity of adequate clearance and excretion of antibiotics as part of aging, since these factors determine drug accumulation and hence the risk of toxicity. Therefore, it is pertinent to develop antibiotic optimization strategies designed with an eye to the peculiar characteristics of the elderly and above all, based on the pharmacokinetic and pharmacodynamic principles [28-30] as well as the most recent advances in pharmacogenetics [31].

The increasing and indiscriminate use of antibiotics has increased bacterial resistance and gives rise to even more resistant strains and hence, therapeutic failures. Such condition could be avoided if antibiotic therapeutic management is based on pharmacokinetic and pharmacodynamic knowledge that promotes beneficial bactericidal concentrations that are within the therapeutic range with sustained effect for each antibiotic [32]. In this context, Van Bambeke and Tulkens [33] showed three important predictors on which the clinical efficacy of the antibiotics are based:

1. The proportion of maximum peak concentration (Cmax) with minimum inhibiting concentration (MIC) i.e., Cmax/MIC

2. The proportion of the area under the curve (AUC) in 24 hours with the minimum inhibiting concentration i.e., AUC(24 hours)/MIC; and
3. The time in which the concentration exceeds the minimum inhibiting concentration (T ≥ MIC).

They sustained that for aminoglycosides and fluoroquinolones, the principal factors for their efficacy depend on the proportion of Cmax/MIC and AUC(24h)/MIC. However, for conventional β-lactamics and macrolides, their efficacy depends on T ≥ MIC while antibiotics whose effects depend on low or weak concentrations are principally related with the quotient AUC 24h)/MIC. The application of these criteria would help in improving the safety and efficacy of the antibiotics in order to prevent bacterial resistance.

Rybak [34] showed that the pharmacokinetic profile of the new generation cephalosporins like cefepime whose activity is against $gram^+$ and $gram^-$ bacteria has been extensively studied not only in adults but also in the elderly, particularly in the later where the elimination is compromised. It was shown in that work that in seven pharmacokinetic studies reported in this cephalosporin (cefepime) that its disposition with respect to linearity, renal excretion and low protein bond is similar to other cephalosporins. On the other part, the work of Riccobene et al. [35] reported thatparenteral ~~(ceftaroline fosfamil)~~ indicated for acute infections of the skin and bacterial pneumonia showed bactericidal activity against $gram^+$ germs including *Staphyloccocus aureus* resistant to methicillin and *Streptococcus pneumoniae* as well as moderately altered pharmacokinetic in the elderly compared with young adults. They attributed this to altered renal function in the elderly. However, they found that the pharmacokinetic of this drug varied with different grades of renal damage. For this reason, they recommended dose adjustment in patients with moderate to severe renal damage.

None of the third generation cephalosporins as cefotaxime, cefoperazone, ceftriaxone, latamoxef, ceftazidime and cefotetan are appropriate for oral administration since their pharmacokinetic has only been studied in their intravascular route of administration. Nonetheless, ceftriaxone is an exception because of its longer half-life elimination (about 8 hr). The other cephalosporins have half-life of elimination range between 1.5 to 2.5 hr. The pharmacokinetic of some cephalosporins can witness modifications in newborns and elderly patients [36]. In such cases, a close monitoring, depending on their pharmacokinetic characteristics, is required.

Pharmacokinetics of Trimethoprim in Elderly and Young Adults

The combination of trimethoprim-sulfamethoxazole mainly for the treatment of infections by gram negative bacteria is widely used since 1968 [37-38]. Its pharmacological activity [39], pharmacokinetics [40, 41] and side effects [42, 43], have been studied in adults. However, there is little information available for geriatric [44] and pediatric populations [45] and even less for newborns. [46] Despite its widespread clinical use in the elderly, the effect of aging on their pharmacokinetics and pharmacodynamics is poorly understood [4, 6, 44]. Hence, one of the main reasons for carrying out this study in adults and elderly Mexicans was to provide scientific basis for designing optimal dosage regimens for trimethoprim-sulfamethoxazole. To carry out the work, the approval of National Institute of Science and Technology-Integral Development of Family (INCYTAS-DIF) bioethics committee of Mexico was sought and obtained.

In the study, nine elderly females with aged between 72 and 90 years were recruited. Their body weight ranged from 36.5 to 78.6 kilograms and their total size was 1.26 to 1.53 meters while their body surface area was 1.11 to 1.61 square meters. Moreover, 8 young healthy voluntary adults (5 females and 3 males) with ages between 25 and 43 years, body weight range was from 45-81 kilograms, height and body surface area 1.44 to 1.74 meters and 1.33 to 1.95 square meters respectively were included as control group.

Prior to 12-hour fast, each person received a single oral dose of 160 mg trimethoprim and 800 mg sulfamethoxazole (two tablets of "Bactrim" Roche Laboratories, containing 80 mg of trimethoprim and 400 mg sulfamethoxazole each). Two hours after drug administration, a light breakfast was given to all participants. Thereafter, there was no dietary restriction neither were there other drug application before or during the study. 0.3 milliliter blood samples were collected prior to medication and subsequent to this at 15, 30, 45 and 60 minutes, 1.52, 3, 4, 6, 8, 12 and 27 hr. By centrifugation, serum was obtained and frozen until analysis. Trimethoprim in serum was quantified by using Schwartz´ spectrofluorometric method [47] after its validation in our laboratory.

The area under the curve of serum concentration versus time (AUC) was calculated using trapezoidal rule. The elimination rate constant (Kel) was obtained by the method of least squares linear regression using the data of the natural logarithm of the serum concentration versus time of the elimination phase. The absorption rate constant (Kab) and distribution (α) were calculated using the method of waste. The half-lives of absorption ($t\frac{1}{2}ab$), distribution

($t\frac{1}{2}$dist) and elimination ($t\frac{1}{2}$el) were calculated by standard procedures [48]. The choice of the pharmacokinetic model of one or two compartments that best suits experienced data was conducted based on the criteria of Akaike [49].

RESULTS

A comparison of the biological variables among the elderly and young adults in relation to body weight, showed no statistically significant difference although, the median is higher in young adults. However, at 5% statistical confidence level, the height and body surface showed statistically significant differences.

When the pharmacokinetic parameters of young adults with those obtained in the group of elders are compared, AUC (0 to ∞ time), the half-life of elimination and the half-life of absorption are found to be larger in the elderly, while the medians of the elimination rate constant (Kel) and absorption (Kab) are greater in young adults. All differences are found to be statistically significant at 0.05 confidence level. In cases where the best model is the open two compartments, the values for the constant rate of distribution and the half-life of distribution showed no significant differences between young adults and the elderly.

Although, the absorption rate constant is lower in the elderly than in younger adults, peak serum concentrations were similar in both groups and above the reported (0.2 μg/mL) [50] inhibitory concentration. In six of the nine elderly, the concentrations close to 1.0 μg/mL were found twelve hours after the administration of trimethoprim while the same concentration was observed in only one of the young adults at the same time.

At present, it is not possible to explain the causes of interindividual variation. Associations between the demographic characteristics (age, weight, height and body surface area) and pharmacokinetic parameters do not seem to be proper, since biological values in both young adults and the elderly tend to cluster at the extremes of the distribution and virtually absent in the middle part of the distribution.

The pharmacokinetics of trimethoprim were adjusted to an open one-compartment model set at 64% for seniors and 38% for adults, and to open two compartments set at 32% for seniors and 62% for young adults who participated in the study. Table 1 shows the pharmacokinetic parameters of the elderly and adults in this study as well as those reported for adults [41, 44] and the elderly.

Table 1. Pharmacokinetic parameters of trimethoprim in the adult and the elderly

	AUC(μg/mL/hr.)	$t_{1/2\,(h)}$	Kab (h^{-1})	α (h^{-1})
Adults (median)	33.86	14.11	1.661	0.539
Elderly (median)	53.55	19.69	0.738	0.630
Literature adults (average)	43.5	11.33	0.726	0.616
Literature elderly	24.83	10.31	1.0756	-

AUC= Area Under Curve, $t_{1/2}$el= Half life of elimination, Kab = Absorption rate constant, α= Distribution rate constant.

Table 2. Initial and Maintenance Dose, and Dosing Interval of trimethoprim

	Initial dose	Maintenance dose	Dosing Interval
Young people	5 tab	2 tab	12 hr
Elderly	4 tab	1 tab	12 hr

The values determined for adults are comparable with those reported in the literature for area under the curve, elimination half-life and constant rate of distribution. The absorption rate constant is greater than that reported by Varoquaux et al. [51] and Welling et al. [40].

The values reported for elderly by Naber et al. [44] are not comparable with those obtained in this study since AUC and elimination half-life reported by them are minor and the constant absorption rate is higher. However, it is important to note that in the study of Naber et al., the ages of the participants were between 70 and 76 years, while the ages of the elderly who participated in the present study were between 72 and 90 years.

The processes of absorption and elimination were faster in adults than in the elderly and so, the dosing regimens used for each group were different (Table 2).

The regimen designed for adults is the same as that reported in the literature while that for the elderly is half the recommended maintenance dose.

Table 3. Pharmacokinetic parameters of trimethoprim in young adults and the elderly

Pharmacokinetic Parameters	Young Adults	Elderly
AUC	-	+
Kel	+	-
tl/2el	-	+
Kab	+	-
tl/2ab	-	+

+ increased, - decreased.

Due to the variability found in the pharmacokinetic parameters in both elderly and adults, the best option is to individualize the regimen whenever possible and titrate it to the pharmaceutical presentations available. In summary, the main findings are shown in Table 3.

It is important to emphasize that for the variability found in the half-lives of elimination for the elderly and young adults, it is recommended to individualize the dosing regimen and this would help to reduce the risk of toxicity.

In Table 4, the pharmacokinetic findings in the elderly, its implications and our recommended modifications based on the result of this study are summarized.

Table 4. Pharmacokinetic changes and its clinic implications

Pharmacokinetic findings in the elderly	Implications	Modified regimen in our study
Absorption is delayed elderly>adults Delayed elimination elderly>adults Plasma concentration predicted elderly>adults	Accumulation of the drug in the body and higher risk of toxicity.	1. Reduce the recommended dose for adult (160 mg every 12 hours) to the half. 2. If the dose of 160 mg is maintained, the administration should be at interval of 24 hours.

REFERENCES

[1] Aparasu RR, Mort JR. Prevalence, correlates, and associated outcomes of potentially inappropriate psychotropic use in the community-dwelling elderly. *Am. J. Geriatr. Pharmacother*. 2004;2 (2):102-111.

[2] Naugler CT, Brymer C, Stolee P, Arcese ZA. Development and validation of an improved prescribing in the elderly tool. *Can. J. Clin. Pharmacol.* 2000; 7(2): 103-107.

[3] Huber M, Blumberg A, Chatterjee S, Haenisch B, Schlosser-Weber G, Broich K. Drug safety: challenge in an aging society. *Nervenarzt*2014; 85(11):1352-62.

[4] Mangoni AA, Jackson SHD. Age-related changes in pharmacokinetics and pharmacodynamics: basic principles and practical applications. *Br J Clin Pharmacol*. 2004; 57(1):6-14.

[5] Klotz U. Pharmacokinetics and drug metabolism in the elderly. *Drug Metab Rev*.2009; 41(2):67-76.

[6] Noreddin AM, El-Khatib W, Haynes V. Optimal dosing design for antibiotic therapy in the elderly: a pharmacokinetic and pharmacodynamic perspective. *Recent Pat Antiinfect Drug Discov*. 2008; 3(1):45-52.

[7] Leikola E, Vartia KO. On penicillin levels in young and geriatric subjects.*J Gerontol*. 1957;12(1):48-52.

[8] Vartia KO, Leikola E. Serum levels of antibiotics in young and old subjects following administration of dihydrostreptomycin and tetracycline. *J Gerontol*.1960; 15:392-4.

[9] Bohr V, Rasmussen N, Hansen B, Kjersem H, Jessen O, Johnsen N, Kristensen HS. 875 cases of bacterial meningitis: diagnostic procedures and the impact of preadmission antibiotic therapy. Part III of a three-part series. *J Infect*. 1983; 7(3):193-202.

[10] Simon N, Décaudin B, Lannoy D, Odou MF, De Broucker M, Barthélémy C, Poret E, Dubreuil L, Odou P. Impact of infusion method on amikacin serum levels in humans. *Pulm Pharmacol Ther*. 2010; 23 (4):324-6.

[11] Boss GR. Age-Related Physiological Changes and Their Clinical Significance. *West J Med*. 1981; 135(6): 434-440.

[12] Gardner ID. The Effect of Aging on Susceptibility to Infection. *Clin Infect Dis*. 1980; 2 (5): 801-810.

[13] Pillai SK, Eliopoulos GM, Moellering RC., Jr Section E: anti-infective therapy: principles of anti-infective therapy. In: Mandell GL, Bennett

JE, Dolin R, editors, eds. *Mandell, Douglas, and Bennett's Principles and Practice of Infectious Diseases*. Vol. 17th ed. Philadelphia, PA: Churchill Livingstone/Elsevier; 2010.

[14] Ginaldi L, De Martinis M,D, Ostilio A, Marini L, Loreto MF, Quaglino D. Immunological changes in the elderly. *Aging* (Milano).1999;11(5): 281-6.

[15] Venjatraman JT, Fernandes G. Exercise, immunity and aging. *Aging* (Milano).1997; 9(1-2):42-56.

[16] Blomberg BB, and Frasca D. Quantity, not quality, of antibody response decreased in the elderly. *J Clin Invest*. 2011; 121(8): 2981-2983.

[17] Riley RL. Impaired B lymphopoiesis in old age: a role for inflammatory B cells?. *Immunol Res*. 2013;57(1-3):361-9.

[18] Asín-Prieto E, Rodríguez-Gascón A, Isla A. Applications of the pharmacokinetic/pharmacodynamic (PK/PD) analysis of antimicrobial agents. *J Infect Chemother*. 2015; 21(5):319-29.

[19] Yoshikawa TT. Antimicrobial Therapy for the Elderly Patient. *J Am Geriatr Soc*. 1990; 38 (12): 1353-1372.

[20] Lewis DA, Reeves DS. Antibiotics at the extremes of age: choices and constraints. *J Antimicrob Chemother*. 1994;34 Suppl. A:11-8.

[21] Ljungberg B and Nilsson-Ehle I. Pharmacokinetics of Antimicrobial Agents in the Elderly. *Rev Infect Dis*. 1987; 9(2):250-64.

[22] Russo M, Iasimone L, Ambrosino E. Antibiotic therapy in the elderly; features and problems. *Infez Med*. 2002;10(4): 204-12.

[23] Lamp KC, Freeman CD, Klutman NE, Lacy MK. Pharmacokinetics and pharmacodynamics of the nitroimidazole antimicrobials. *Clin Pharmacokinet*. 1999;36(5):353-73.

[24] Cios A, Wyska E, Szymura-Oleksiak J, Grodzicki T. Population pharmacokinetic analysis of ciprofloxacin in the elderly patients with lower respiratory tract infections. *Exp Gerontol*. 2014; 57:107-13.

[25] Advenier C, Saint-Aubin A, Gobert C, Houin G, Albengres E, Tillement JP. Pharmacokinetics of isoniazid in the elderly. *Br J Clin Pharmacol*. 1980; 10(2):167-9.

[26] Stalam M, and kaye D. Antibiotic agent in the elderly. *Infect Dis Clin North Am*. 2000; 14(2):357-69.

[27] Posner JD. Particular problems of antibiotic use in the elderly. *Geriatrics*. 1982; 37(8):49-54.

[28] Noreddin AM, Haynes V. Use of pharmacodynamic principles to optimise dosage regimens for antibacteria lagents in the elderly. *Drug aging*. 2007;24(4):275-92.

[29] Bengt Ljungberg and Ingrid Nilsson-Ehle. Pharmacokinetics of Antimicrobial Agents in the Elderly. *Reviews of Infectious Diseases.* 1987;9(2):250-264.

[30] Hutchison LC, O'Brien CE. Changes in pharmacokinetics and pharmacodynamics in the elderly patient. *J Pharm Prac* 2007;20:4-12.

[31] Bright DR, Calinski DM, and Kisor DF. Pharmacogenetic considerations in the elderly patient. *Consult Pharm* 2015;30(4):228-39.

[32] Smith SV, Gould IM. Optimization of antibiotic dosing schedules in the light of increasing antibiotic resistance. *Expert Rev Anti Infec Ther.* 2004; 2(2).227-34.

[33] Van Bambeke F, Tulkens PM. Macrolides:pharmacokinetics and pharmacodynamics. *Int J Antimicrob Agents.* 2001, 18 Suppl. 1:S17-23.

[34] Rybak M. The pharmacokinetic profile of a new generation of parenteral cephalosporin. *Am J Med* 1996 june 24; 100(6A):39S-44S.

[35] Riccobene T, Jakate A y Rank D. A series of pharmacokinetic studies of ceftaroline fosamil in select populations: normal subjects, healthy elderly subjects with renal impairment or end-stage renal disease requiring hemodialysis. *J Clin Pharmacol* 2014; 54(7): 742-52.

[36] Balant L, Dayer P, Auckenthaler R. Clinical pharmacokinetic of the third generation cephalosporins. *Clin Pharmacokinet.* 1985;10(2):101-43.

[37] Bushby SR, Hitchings GH. Trimethoprim, a sulphonamide potentiator. *Br J Pharmacol Chemother.* 1968; 33(1):72-90.

[38] Hughes DT, Drew CD, Johnson TB, Jarvis JD. Trimethoprim and sulphamethoxazole in the treatment of chronic chest infections. *Chemotherapy.* 1969;14(3):151-7.

[39] Bushby SR. Trimethoprim-sulfamethoxazole: *in vitro* microbiological aspects. *J Infect Dis.* 1973;128:Suppl:442-62.

[40] Welling PG, Craig WA, Amidon GL, Kunin CM. Pharmacokinetics of trimethoprim and sulfamethoxazole in normal subjects and in patients with renal failure. *J Infect Dis.* 1973; 128:Suppl:556-66.

[41] Craig WA, Kunin CM. Trimethoprim-sulfamethoxazole: pharmacodynamic effects of urinary pH and impaired renal function. Studies in humans. *Ann Intern Med.* 1973; 78(4):491-7.

[42] Frisch JM. Clinical experience with adverse reactions to trimethoprim-sulfamethoxazole. *J Infect Dis.* 1973; 128:Suppl:607-12.

[43] Jenkins GC, Hughes DT, Hall PC. A haematological study of patients receiving long-term treatment with trimethoprim and sulphonamide. *J Clin Pathol.* 1970;23(5): 392-6.

[44] Naber K, Vergin H, Weigand W. Pharmacokinetics of co-trimoxazole and co-tetroxazine in geriatric patients. *Infection*. 1981; 9(5):239-43.

[45] Wilfert CM: Trimethoprim-sulfamethoxazole in children: pharmacokinetics and clinical studies. *J Infect Dis*. 1973; 128 (Suppl.): 613-617.

[46] Springer C, Eyal F, and Michel J. Pharmacology of trimetoprim-sulfamethoxazole in newborn Infants. *J Pediatr*. 1982; 100 (4): 647-650.

[47] Schwartz DE, Koechlin BA, and Weinfel RE. Spectrofluorometric method for the determination of trimethoprim in body fluids. *Chemotherapy*. 1969; 14(Suppl.):22-9.

[48] Milo Gibaldi M y Donald Perrier. 1982. Farmacocinética. Editorial Reverté S.A., Salamanca, pp. 287-298.

[49] Yamaoka K, Nakagawa T, and Uno T.: Application of Akalke's Information criterion (AIC) in the evaluation of linear pharmacokinetics equations. *J Pharmacokin Biopharm*. 1978; 6(2):165-175.

[50] Clinical and Laboratory Standards Institute (CLSI). Performance Standards for Antimicrobial Susceptibility Testing; Twenty-third Informational Supplement, CLSI document M100-S23. CLSI document M100-S23, Clinical and Laboratory Standards Institute, 950 West Valley Road, Suite 2500, Wayne, Pennsylvania 19087, US, 2013.

[51] Varoquaux O, Lajoie D, Gobert C, Cordonnier P, Ducreuzet C, Pays M, Advenier C. Pharmacokinetics of the trimethoprim-sulphamethoxazole combination in the elderly. *Br J Clin Pharmacol*. 1985; 20(6): 575-581.

In: Optimization of Drug Prescribing in Elderly ISBN: 978-1-63484-879-4
Editors: Juárez O. H. and Lares A. I.

Chapter 11

PATTERNS OF DRUG CONSUMPTION IN OLDER PERSONS

Belén Juárez Tapia[1,*], David Calderón Guzmán[2] and Hugo Juárez Olguín[3]

[1]Laboratorio de Farmacología, Instituto Nacional de Pediatría, Mexico City
[2]Laboratorio de Neurociencias, Instituto Nacional de Pediatría, México
[3]Laboratorio de Farmacología, Instituto Nacional de Pediatría, Mexico City, Mexico, and Departamento de Farmacología, Facultad de Medicina, Universidad Nacional Autónoma de México, México

ABSTRACT

The elder population suffers higher number of diseases than younger population. Therefore, the consumption of drugs is higher in this population than in the rest of the populations. A recent study made in USA shows that proximately 77% of individuals older than 65 years old consume at least one drug. Even though that these people represent 12% of total population, their rate of drug consumption corresponds to 30% of all the drugs used in that country. Other reports indicate that this population consume between 1.5 and 4.2 drugs at the same time. This

* Corresponding author: Belén Juárez Tapia, Laboratorio de Farmacología, InstitutoNacional de Pediatría. AvenidaImán # 1, 3er piso, Col Cuicuilco, CP 04530, Mexico D.F, Mexico.e-mail: mcr_balmar@hotmail.com.

represents a big financial cost and apart from this, the inherent risks of polypharmacy related with factors of aging increase and this might lead to possible apparition of adverse effects, which can be severe for health. In the present study, we describe the pattern of drug consumption based on previous reports made in elderly Mexican population in comparison with investigations made in other countries. In this regard, it was found that drugs that are mostly consumed are those used in cardiovascular and in central nervous system problems as well as antiinflammatory and analgesic drugs. However, the conclusion in both studies points to the necessity of implementing public health politics directed to improving the use of medicaments in the elderly population based on a correct prescription, compliance evaluation and avoidance of simultaneous use of multidrug. The implementation of this kind of politics would significantly help to improve the health of the elderly people and eliminate the risk of bad or incorrect use of drugs.

INTRODUCTION

As people get older, their pattern of drug consumption changes. Driven by the desire to treat and control conditions resulting from aging process, the elderly people are proned to consume more medicines. However, the better the prescription and the more adequate is the treatment compliance, the better is the efficacy and the safety of the drug. Older people have a high risk of toxicity with medications, since four out of five people over 75 take at least one medication and 36% of them take four or more medicines at the same time. Human body, during the aging process may be more susceptible to side effects of medicines [1]. Older adults with multiple diseases often take many drugs at the same time, which increases the risk of toxicity or therapeutic failure by drug interactions. Aging ailments as osteoarthritis, visual disorders and neurodegenerative diseases among others, may promote unnecessary consumption of medicines some of which are bought out of the counter [2].

These problems are exacerbated because of non-compliance to medical advice and in some cases, the expiration date is likely disregarded. The problem is even greater when the person does not have a family or anyone to monitor his/her treatment compliance [3].

In view of all the aforementioned points, it is important and necessary to know the pharmacoepidemiology of drugs prescribed to older people and to ensure their correct usage.

SITUATION IN MEXICO

In Mexico, as in many other countries, the phenomenon of demographic and epidemiological transition indicates an increase in the older population [4]. The population people over 60 years old in Mexico in 1964 represented 5.6%. In 1990, it was increased to 6.14%, and by the year 2000, it was 7,2% (Figure 1).

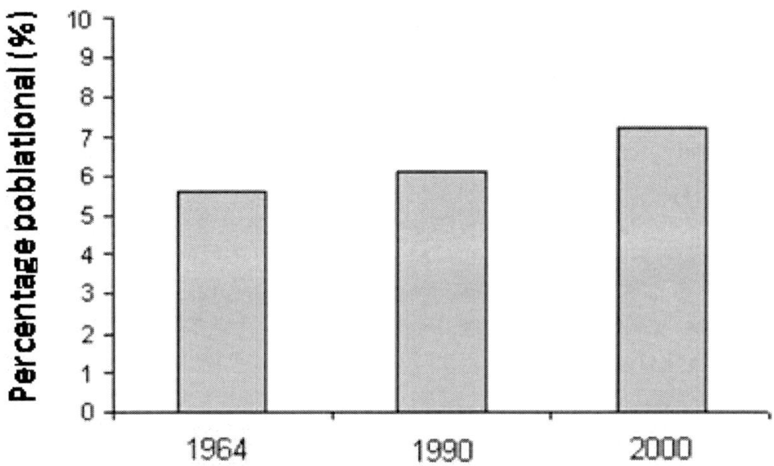

Figure 1. Percentage of people over 60years old in Mexico in 1964, 1990 and 2000.

The obviousness of increasing life expectance as the years pass is clear in the population not only of Mexico but also worldwide. This tantamount to a decrease in mortality of the elderly people and an increase in the appearance of new diseases and a surge of multiple and chronic degenerative diseases. This situation is already present for some years in Mexico and has been generating a high and complex use of drugs procured both by prescription and over the counter. Undoubtedly, this poses difficult problems for aged people and the health sectors as a whole.

The older people are more predisposed to illness than the young ones. Hence the former consume significantly more medications. A study in the United States indicates that about 77% of the people aged 65 or more, take at least one medication and although, they represent only 12% of the population, they consume about 30% of all the drugs sold in pharmacies. On average, the number of drugs that this population receives at the same time varies between 1.5 and 4.2. Besides being expensive, multiple consumptions represent a major clinical risk, since the physical deterioration in these patients increases the risk of adverse effects [5, 6]. The risk also depends on the specific combinations of medicines [7].

Women generally consume more drugs than men, although it has been observed that at older ages, this association is lost. However, it is possible that women are more susceptible to the adverse effects as they experience greater decrease in body mass and therefore major changes in basal metabolic rate [8].

Consuming large amounts of medicines can affect the quality of life, that is why physicians must seriously consider the basis of drug prescription even when these are aimed at improving the quality of life. Side effects that may occur when medicines are taken be it prescribed or over the count, have been linked to conditions that can lead to disability in the aged and as a causal factor, involving about 10% of all hospitalizations.

Recent studies have reported that inappropriate use of medicines could cause about 25% of hospital admissions and that the risk of an adverse effect increases with the number of drugs prescribed [9, 10]. The increased use does not only have a medical history, but also social and cultural. Developed countries have in general a higher older population, but even in those who are under development as is the case of Mexico, increased attention to degenerative diseases and the development of therapeutically more effective drugs have been observed. Higher availability of drugs leads to larger consumption. In developed countries, most medications are only available by prescription and dispensed by pharmacists. This means that the therapeutic practices of physicians and pharmacists regulate their use. However, psychological and social factors have a major impact in the patterns usage: living alone, feelings of loneliness and depressive symptoms have been associated with high consumption of certain drugs.

A new behaviour has occurred among the older ones. This lies on the consumption of vitamins and trace elements usually by the high social classes and those who are more concerned about their health (Table 1). Inappropriate prescription of these compounds for the older population has recently taken a new dimension and it represents a big problem, although its magnitude is still unknown.

In México, a large proportion of the drugs for seniors are provided free of charge. The patterns of prescriptions are multiple. Most of the time, the drugs are "self-indicated" or "indicated" by the drug store attendant or pharmacist. Other sources of prescription are a family member and a neighbour or friend who usually bases their prescription on past experiences with the drug or copied from their previous visit to a physician. Another pattern is when a physician prescribes at the patient's own request. For this reason, it is inconceivable medication out of prescription or over the count as in other countries. In countries like Mexico, no distinction is made between prescribed and consumed, since it is most likely that the consumed are prescribed, be it either specialist prescriptions or quark prescriptions - non-specialist indications. Thus, patients take medications even when small disturbances are experienced [11].

Table 1. Commonly prescribed nutrients in two nursing homes for older people in Mexico City

	Men n=135	Women n=227	Total n =362
Calcium	1.5	6.2	4.5
Protein	0.0	0.9	0.5
Iron	2.2	0.9	1.4
Thiamine	0.0	0.9	0.5
Pyridoxine	0.7	0.0	0.3
Cyanocobalamin	0.0	0.4	0.3
Potassium	0.9	0.7	0.8

It has been found that in our country, as in other countries, women consume more drugs than men. This is probably because women are more thoughtful or concerned about their health and their perception of pain and its prevalence are higher with more affective and neurological symptoms as memory loss, sadness or insomnia compared with men (Table 2)[12].

Table 2. Commonly prescribed analgesics in two nursing homes for older people in Mexico City

	Men n=135	Women n=227	Total n =362
Non-steroidal anti-inflammatories	8,1	17,6	14,1
Paracetamol	2,9	5,7	4,7
Magnesium dipirone/hyoscine	0,7	2,2	1,7
Codeine-based agents	0,7	2,2	1,7
Tramadol	0,0	2,7	1,7

However, by excluding those who do not consume drugs, the average is generally equal in men than in women. This probably indicates that consumption occurs equally in diseased and symptomatic people, regardless of gender nevertheless, morbidity is more prevalent in women [13].

It was estimated that 40-45% of the aged people do not consume drugs as indicated. This may be even more prevalent with medications indicated for three or four times a day and those that are not consumed daily. It is easier to remember to take one pill indicated for certain days in the week or month. The variable number of dose/drug quantity or amount indicated goes to show the complexities of the regimen [14]. In a study conducted by Arlt et al., a dose/drug ratio of 1:4 was observed and that only 7.3% of the population has consumed regularly prescribed medications. This means that most of the doses contain 4 drugs. Therefore, the rate at which the drug and dosage prescribed is what counts for optimal adherence to treatment.

DISEASE RELATED WITH DRUG CONSUMPTION

In recent studies made by our research group in some nursing homes in Mexico City, including two asylums, one particular and the other government-based (Mundet and DIF, respectively), we found a distribution of therapeutic groups where the greatest consumption was observed for drugs to treat cardiovascular diseases, central nervous system and analgesic/anti-inflammatory drugs, reflecting a higher prevalence of some diseases in the older people (Tables 3, 4, 5, 6, 7).

Table 3. Commonly prescribed cardiovascular drugs in two nursing homes for older people in Mexico City

	Men n = 135	Women n = 227	Total n = 362
Antihypertensive	37,6	44,2	41,8
Diuretics	10,2	13,7	12,5
Digoxin	4,4	5,3	5,0
Other antiarrhythmic drugs	0,0	1,8	1,1
Anticlotting agents (no aspirin)	6,6	1,3	3,3
Aspirin	9,4	12,3	11,3
Venodilators	4,3	9,2	7,5
Peripheral vasodilators	5,8	6,6	6,3
Beta-blockers	1,5	1,8	1,7

Table 4. Commonly prescribed drugs for the treatment of respiratory (A) and digestive (B) illnesses, in two nursing homes for older people in Mexico City

(A)

	Men n=135	Women n=227	Total n =362
Bronchodilators	7,2	1,8	3,9
Anti-flu	5,1	3,5	4,1
Oxygen	0,7	0,0	0,3

(B)

	Men n=135	Women n=227	Total n =362
Laxatives	2,2	2,6	2,5
Alkalis	6,7	4,9	5,6
Antihistaminic H2	11,1	3,5	6,4

Table 5. Commonly prescribed drugs acting on the central nervous system in two nursing homes for older people in Mexico City

	Men n=135	Women n=227	Total n =362
Antidepressants	1,5	9,7	6,6
Benzodiazepines and novel hypnotics	8,1	22,9	17,4
Neuroleptics	3,7	5,7	5,0
Brain vasodilators	13,3	26,0	21,3
Anti-vertigo	0,0	2,2	1,4
Anti-convulsants	3,0	0,5	1,4
Anti-parkinson	0,0	0,9	0,5

Table 6. Commonly prescribed drugs acting on the endocrine system (metabolism) in two nursing homes for older people in Mexico City

	Men n=135	Women n=227	Total n =362
Hypolipaemiants	8,1	9,7	9,1
Oral antidiabetics	9,4	13,7	12,1
Hypouricaemiants	0,7	0,9	0,8
Insulin	1,5	2,6	2,2
Thyroid hormones	0,7	0,0	0,3
Progestagens	0,7	0,0	0,3
Gonadotropins	0,7	0,0	0,3
Oral corticosteroids	1,5	1,3	1,4
Ointments	0,7	0,4	0,6
Inhaled	2,2	0,9	1,4

Table 7. Other drugs prescribed in two nursing homes for older people in Mexico City

Anti-allergy/anti-histaminic H1	4,4	1,3	2,5
Calcitonin	0,0	3,5	2,2
Eye drops	4,3	1,8	2,8
Drugs aimed at treating prostate benign hypertrophy	5,8	0,0	2,5
Antibiotics	5,1	2,7	3,6

THE MEXICAN PROFILE

To analyse these data, we used the ATC classification level 1. It is noteworthy that some of these results have not yet been published. Some differences related to the date of the study can be noticed, for example, the use of diuretics (12.5%) was lower than others made in the 80s (36%), before the appearance of new antihypertensive drugs [15,16]. High consumption of cerebral vasodilators, of dubious therapeutic efficacy can be explained by the high prevalence of subjective complaints of memory loss, especially in women in most populations. In another Spanish population sample reported by Valderrama et al. [17], the use of these drugs amounted to a third of the population studied. One third of the older people consume multiple drugs (four or more medications), a fact that has also been observed in other studies by Marin et al. [18].

Measures that may have a positive effect in reducing polypharmacy are:

1. Reducing the prevalence of these and other drugs with low therapeutic value.
2. Establishment of moderate exercise.
3. Implementation of healthy eating habits and
4. The application of alternative therapeutic activities such as meditation and relaxation.

Some gender differences in the types of drugs frequently consumed by elderly people reside on agents targeted to the central nervous system and pain for women and for men, drugs for respiratory problems. This reflects the gender distribution of certain health problems [19]. However, it is risky to make a projection of the diseases that affect men and women by the type of drug consumed; e.g., in Table 4 there is more use of antiacids in men than in women, but there is no evidence that there are differences of this disease among both sexes.

The use of antipsychotics has been studied, however, the problem goes far beyond this category of drugs. The type of medication used by older people is closely related to their chronic conditions. [20]. For example, morphine is consumed to relieve pain, and barbiturates to treat insomnia. This kind of use is justified by the loss of physical and psychological faculties and the proximity of death, resulting in symptoms of depression, anxiety, distress, so that opioids and depressants are the most consumed (Table 5) [21, 22]. Benzodiazepines are often prescribed and those who take them on many occasions continue their use indefinitely. [23]Drugs that can cause physical dependence should be restricted to prescription under medical treatment and the use outside prescription or at the self-administration should be considered as drugs of abuse [24].

Health Requirements

The Ministry of Health of Mexico in 1993, through the Department of Epidemiology, held the Second National Survey of Addictions (ENA 93) [4]. The objectives of the survey were a) to gather information at the regional and national levels on the prevalence and abuse of snuffing, alcohol, opioids, central nervous system depressants and other depressants, stimulants, marijuana, inhalants, hallucinogens, heroin, opium and cocaine derivatives; b) to identify potential risk factors and problems associated with their consumption; c) to identify attitudes and values towards the use of different addictive substances [25]. The purpose of ENA 93 was however, not to provide specific information on the older population in the country. This initial analysis shows the drug consumption picture and how it should be more extensively studied at both national and regional levels. Moreover, it revealed the demographic characteristics of the older population who consume medically prescribed drugs as drugs of abuse. Due to the characteristics of this epidemiological revision, ethical authorization is not required, but data from population is reserved.

This survey provided an opportunity to know the characteristics of antipsychotic drugs abuse by the older population. It is noteworthy that the selected sample was stratified by region and sex, and only in the urban population were people between 60 and 65 years old considered, which limits the possible inference from the results. Demographic differences found in XI Census regarding the occupational and educational population distribution in both rural and urban areas are simply census data. There is a clear difference in the use of drug between men and women. As previously mentioned, women consume more drugs than men. The aforesaid can be supported by the fact that there are older women than men and because women use medical services more frequently than men.

In our country, Mexico City has the largest concentration of hospitals and health centres. On this basis, it is expected that drug consumption in the city should be higher than in the rest of the country. However, the results were rather different, since some provinces (Aguascalientes, Colima, Jalisco, Nayarit, Zacatecas, Chihuahua, Durango and Coahuila) recorded higher sales of drugs than in the capital. This can be explained by the method of selecting the sample, which was lower in Mexico City. Moreover, the sample did not specifically and statistically represent the population of 60-65 years old. However, since 12% of the older people in the country live in such regions, these results were expected [26].

DISCUSSION

Statistics concerning the intake of drug for treatment of ailments in any part of the world should take into consideration such factors as chronic disease morbidity, demographic characteristics, level of education, occupation and the level of income among others. The ENA 93 survey showed that the demographic characteristics of consumers of therapeutic drugs are different from those of the surveyed population. Education and occupation are undoubtedly important factors that could influence drug consumption pattern. People with higher levels of formal education and professional-type activities consume more drugs. This lies on the fact that procurement of expert prescription implies an expenses not only in medical consultation, which is often private, but sometimes also in the drug itself as demonstrated by the same survey and consequently, people with more education and better jobs have better access to many medicines. The above assumption does not attempt to link the level of income with the rate of drug consumption. It is just an inference that could be made since the survey did not provide data directly linking income with consumption.

A low proportion of users (15%) who took drugs without prescription were identified. This is different from Spain where 47% was found. Nevertheless, the use of multiple drugs at the same time is dangerous and should not be permitted since the side effects which could arise out of it may jeopardize the health of the user apart from taking him or her to dependency to such substances. It was reported that about 10% of older people take drugs recommended by others quark prescription, and more than 20% take non-prescription drugs. It is important to mention the need to encourage the medical community to improve the monitoring of adequate intake of these drugs.

In Spain, García-Fernández noted that 24% of subjects in a sample took CNS depressants; with benzodiazepines being the most frequently used (62.3%) [27]. According to the ENA 93, 18.7% of the people use CNS depressants, however, the true prevalence in Mexico varies between 8.1 and 30.6%.

The above results indicate the need for specific studies to address the particular problems of the older people through their identification and to seek for alternative solutions to problems as the failure of medical treatment, which can be in the form of overdose and abuse, neglect and alteration of doses and schedules.

Some older patients with acute conditions take excessive amount of medication when they feel discomfort, believing that this will help them recover faster. This excessive consumption is related to the adverse effects of drugs [28, 29]. Also, remembering to take their medication is a common problem and is more common in subjects taking multiple drugs. In the elderly, it is essential to be alert to the diseases that occur at the same time to avoid inappropriate administration of multiple pharmaceutical agents, the potential risk of dependency and abuse. It is necessary to conduct more research that would help to understand the characteristics of the use of medical drugs by the population over 65 years, the use of multiple medications and their association with the presence of adverse effects.

In men, the proportion that used daily medications and the average of these medications increased with age, but not in women, where the largest proportion of consumers and higher average was found in the intermediate age group. In some studies, differences in drug use between men and women are shortened in those older than 85 years. It is difficult to determine whether the proportion of medicines consumed with no fixed pattern, i.e., those medicines that people consume only when certain symptoms appear (20%), is high or not. In other studies, only 10% of the population consumed drugs when the need arose, but this included a combined sample of subjects admitted to nursing homes and individuals attended in health centres. So, there must surely be people sicker or very sick and are more dependent on regular consumption of drugs [30]. Although medications must be prescribed by a doctor, taking certain therapeutic agents when the need arises and with medical advice, is not only a recommendable practice, but also for the self-care of certain chronic diseases such as degenerative joint disease or chronic obstructive disease of the lung. The high proportion of subjects taking chronic medication is justified by the high prevalence of chronic diseases in the older people.

As final considerations, errors of prescription, over-the-counter consumption, polypharmacy and increased frequency of adverse events, can be very serious drawbacks of pharmacotherapy in the older population. However, these problems can be minimized and prevented in a large proportion and magnitude by promoting the adoption of healthy habits from an early age. This situation is more important considering that the older population is increasing greatly and that in the future, this might overpower medical supplies, clinics and hospitals specializing in geriatrics. Also, friendly sites that would promote the life of the old aged, such as special seats on public transport, ramps and overpass with elevators and escalators enough to satisfy the entire population of older adults will be required. So, the promotion of health care in young people should be a global priority for public health and preventive medicine.

It must be remembered that, as with any medical intervention, the best drug treatment is the one that is not used. The older population is where this guideline should be applied in full. And so, clinicians are required to minimize the prescription of drugs to the old aged and seek alternative measures such as a constant healthy diet, moderate physical activity, naturism and recreational activities.

The chronic use of drugs in Mexican by older people is considerable. It is not far different from other populations because studies have shown it to be very similar consumption.

EXPECTANCE

Regarding the few population-based studies made abroad, any comparison would be risky. The agents most consumed are directed to the cardiovascular system, central nervous system and analgesic/anti-inflammatory drugs, which is an indicator of diseases in the older population in our country. However, it is necessary to carry out more specific studies regarding the patterns of medication use by the older people including the frequency of adverse effects. Furthermore, efforts to encourage the adoption of healthy habits from young age, as well as better use of drugs in the old age are needed in the ambit of correct indication of the drug, good compliance, avoidance of possible polypharmacy to ensure the optimization of drug use in the old aged.

REFERENCES

[1] Borges-Yáñez SA, Gómez-Dantés H. The use of health services for population elder than 60 years in Mexico. *Salud Publica Mexico* 1998; 40: 13-23.

[2] Beynon CM. Drug use and ageing: older people do take drugs!. *Age Ageing* 2009; 38: 8-10.

[3] Kendrick R, Bayne JR. Compliance with prescribed medication by elderly patients. *Can Med Assoc J* 1982; 127: 961-962.

[4] Tapia-Conyer R, Cravioto P, Borges-Yáñez A, De la Rosa B. Medicine consumption in population between 60 and 65 years in Mexico. National Survey of Addictions. 1993. *Salud Publica Mexico* 1996; 38: 458-465.

[5] Gidal BE. Drug absorption in the elderly: biopharmaceutical considerations for the antiepileptic drugs. *Epilepsy Res* 2006; 68 Suppl 1: S65-9.

[6] Conil JM, Georges B, Lavit M. Pharmacokinetics of ceftazidime and cefepime in burn patients: the importance of age and creatinine clearance. *Int J Clin Pharmacol Ther* 2007; 45: 529-538.

[7] Metlay JP. Medication comprehension and safety in older adults. *LDI Issue Brief* 2008; 14: 1-4.

[8] Levine MA, Grootendorst P. Proportion of osteoporotic post-menopausal women at increased risk for upper GI adverse events associated with bisphosphonate therapy. *Pharmacoepidemiol Drug Safety* 2000; 9: 367-370.

[9] Cassidy N, Lee SK, Donegan CF, Tracey JA. Poisoning in older adults: the experience of the national poisons information centre. *Ir Med J* 2008; 101: 268-270.

[10] Haider SI, Johnell K, Weitoft GR, Thorslund M, Fastbom J. The influence of educational level on polypharmacy and inappropriate drug use: a register-based study of more than 600,000 older people. *J Am Geriatr Soc* 2009; 57: 62-69.

[11] Staatz CE, Tett SE. Pharmacokinetic considerations relating to tacrolimus dosing in the elderly. *Drugs Aging* 2005; 22: 541-557.

[12] Pautex S, Vogt-Ferrier N. Management of chronic pain in older persons. *Rev Medical Suisse* 2006; 2: 1629-1630.

[13] Mangoni AA. Cardiovascular drug therapy in elderly patients: specific age-related pharmacokinetic, pharmacodynamic and therapeutic considerations. *Drugs Aging* 2005; 22: 913-941.

[14] Arlt S, Lindner R, Rösler A, von Renteln-Kruse W. Adherence to medication with dementia: predictors and strategies for improvement. *Drugs Aging* 2008; 25: 1033-1047.

[15] Staskin DR. Over active bladder in the elderly: a guide to pharmacological management. *Drugs Aging* 2005; 22: 1013-1928.

[16] Tsuyuki RT, McLean DL, McAlister FA. Management of hypertension in elderly long-term care residents. *Can J Cardiol* 2008; 24: 912-914.

[17] Valderrama E, Rodríguez F, Palacios A, Gabarre P, Pérez del Molino J. Consumption of medicines in elderly: Results of a population study. *Rev Esp Salud Publica* 1998; 72: 209-219.

[18] Marin GH, Cañas M, Homar C, Ylarri E, Pena D, Trebuco H. Use of drugs in elderly attended in a institution from a province of Buenos Aires, Argentina. *Lat Am J Pharm* 2010; 29: 495-503.

[19] Bellia V, Battaglia S, Matera MG, Cazzola M. The use of bronchodilators in the treatment of airway obstruction in elderly patients. *PulmonPharmacolTher* 2006; 19: 311-319.

[20] Weiser ML. Antipsychotics: restraints for the elderly?. *Am J Nurs* 2008; 108: 11.

[21] Perucca E, Berlowitz D, Birnbaum A, et al. Pharmacological and clinical aspects of antiepileptic drug use in the elderly. *Epilepsy Res* 2006; 68 Suppl 1: S49-63.

[22] Leppik IE. Epilepsy in the elderly. *Rev Neurol Dis* 2004; 1 Suppl 1: S44-55.

[23] Hilleret H, Falconnet C, Le Saint L, Perrenoud JJ, Michel JP, Vogt-Ferrier N. Prescribing psychotropic drugs aged 80 and over. *Rev Medical Suisse* 2008; 4: 2405-8.

[24] [24]Allain H, Bentué-Ferrer D, Polard E, Akwa Y, Patat A. Postural instability and consequent falls and hip fractures associated with use of hypnotics in the elderly: a comparative review. *Drugs Aging* 2005; 22: 749-765.

[25] Ministry of Health, National Survey of addictions. Medical drugs. Mexico, D.F. *General Direction of Epidemiology,* SSA, 1994.

[26] Pérez-Guillé G, Camacho-Vieyra A, Toledo-López A, Guillé-Pérez A, Flores-Pérez J. Patterns of drug consumption in relation with the pathologies of elderly Mexican subjects resident in nursing homes. *J Pharmacol Pharm Sci* 2001; 4: 159-166.

[27] García-Fernández J, González-Pérez C, Sánchez MM, Sánchez-Baragaño M, Vega JB, Méndez-Rodríguez M. Psychotropic drugs consumption in erderly. *Rev SanidHigPublica* 1994; 68: 303-310.

[28] Ginsberg G, Hattis D, Russ A, Sonawane B. Pharmacokinetic and pharmacodynamic factors that can affect sensibility to neurotoxic sequelae in elderly individuals. *Environ Health Perspec* 2005; 113: 1243-1249.

[29] Barni S, Cabiddu M, Petrelli F. Toxicity of targeted therapies in elderly patients. *Expert Rev Anticancer Ther* 2008; 8: 1965-1976.

[30] Doucet J. Use of antidiabetic drugs in elderly patients. *Diabetes Metab* 2005; 31: 5S98-5S104.

Editors' Contact Information

Dr. Hugo Juárez Olguín
Email: juarezol@yahoo.com

Dr. Ismael Lares Asseff
CIIDIR, Durango, Mexico
Fax: 5729 6000 (82621)
Email: ismaelares@yahoo.com

Index

#

A

C

D

E

F

I

J

K

L

M

N

Q

R

S

T

U

V

W

Y